Yogic Peace Education

Yogic Peace Education

Theory and Practice

Katerina Standish
and Janine M. Joyce

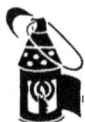

McFarland & Company, Inc., Publishers
Jefferson, North Carolina

LIBRARY OF CONGRESS CATALOGUING-IN-PUBLICATION DATA

Names: Standish, Katerina, author. | Joyce, Janine M., 1965– author.
Title: Yogic peace education : theory and practice / Katerina Standish and Janine M. Joyce.
Description: Jefferson, North Carolina : McFarland & Company, Inc., Publishers, 2018 | Includes bibliographical references and index.
Identifiers: LCCN 2017049561 | ISBN 9781476670010 (softcover : acid free paper) ∞
Subjects: LCSH: Peace—Study and teaching. | Nonviolence—Study and teaching. | Yoga—Philosophy.
Classification: LCC JZ5534 .S75 2018 | DDC 303.6/6071—dc23
LC record available at https://lccn.loc.gov/2017049561

BRITISH LIBRARY CATALOGUING DATA ARE AVAILABLE

ISBN (print) 978-1-4766-7001-0
ISBN (ebook) 978-1-4766-3016-8

© 2018 Katerina Standish and Janine M. Joyce. All rights reserved

No part of this book may be reproduced or transmitted in any form or by any means, electronic or mechanical, including photocopying or recording, or by any information storage and retrieval system, without permission in writing from the publisher.

Front cover image © 2018 iStock

Printed in the United States of America

McFarland & Company, Inc., Publishers
 Box 611, Jefferson, North Carolina 28640
  www.mcfarlandpub.com

Table of Contents

Acknowledgments	vii
Introduction	1

Part I: Peace Education
One—What Is Peace Education?	7
Two—Peace Education as Cultural Nonviolence	29

Part II: Yogic Science
Three—What Is Yoga?	45
Four—Yoga and Life Nourishment	72
Five—Gatherings: Yoga and Groups	92
Six—Learning Peace	115
Toolkit 1: Learning Without Violence	136
Toolkit 2: Living Without Violence	143
Toolkit 3: Loving Without Violence	150

Glossary	157
Appendix: Chakra Coloring Meditation	161
Chapter Notes	171
Bibliography	173
Index	183

Acknowledgments

This book began with a brief, agreeable conversation that drew connections between two previously distinct sub worlds: Yoga and peace education. The Hindu god Ganesh is said to be the "remover of obstacles" and among his powers is the ability to clear a pathway forward or put blocks in front of you when you are going the wrong way! As our way opened up for us like a grand vista of possibility we perceived that we must be going in a favorable direction.

This book manifested without struggle in a creative and compelling manner. During the course of our two distinct lives we have found ourselves returning repeatedly to "things we already know" or knowledge and wisdom "we forgot we had already learned." This is important because among the underpinnings that gird this book is the understanding of unity and interconnectivity in the universe and the sense that self-knowledge is good knowledge and that in order to find self-knowledge you must *look for it*. We had faith that if we were going in the proper direction the wind would be warmly at our backs. This book is where the wind meets the land. We thank our future readers in advance if our journey has proved fruitful and valuable.

Katerina's Acknowledgments

This book would not be possible were it not for the hundreds of students and teachers who shared space (and continue to share space) along my learning journey. I have taught formal and informal Yoga, and peace education for over a decade and I am grateful and honored to be a part of the mindful exchange of wellness that characterizes both Yoga and education for peace. This book was nurtured in the surprisingly fertile underbelly of the planet at the National Centre for Peace and Conflict Studies in Dunedin, New Zealand. I am thankful for the trail of wisdom, hope and joy my work has followed and must mention that this book was sustained through the inspiration, intelligent suggestions, guidance and friendship of numerous individuals, most notably Heather Devere, Douglas Allen, Kevin Clements, Cheryl Duckworth, Laura Finley, Robin Cooper, Dale Snauwaert, Lynne Rienner, Zvi Bekerman, Daniel Bar-Tal, Sean Byrne, Heather Kertyzia and Rhondda Davies. Very special thanks to our anonymous reviewers for their insightful comments and suggestions. I thank my husband Corey and my scrumptious daughter Madelin for buckets of love and wish to express my deep affection and gratitude to Janine Joyce for being such a beautiful, wonderful, challenging, bright and insightful companion on this expedition!

Janine's Acknowledgments

A creative project such as a book often represents the fruit of a long gestation of learning, exploration and discovery. Such is the case here. I would like to honor all my Yogic teachers particularly those based within the Sri Ram Chandra Mission, Chennai, India, and the Rashtriya Sanskrit Vidyapeetha, Tirupathi, India. I am grateful to the Indian Government and the Commonwealth scholarship that allowed me to spend extensive periods of time living on the land and with the peoples of India. The Indian Yogic cultural heritage has been developed by the work of many reputable scientists interested in humanity's consciousness for thousands of years. Our work here is one small leaf on a mighty tree of learning, dedication, sacrifice, inspiration and exploration by thousands of others before us. It is difficult in the context of such a stream of heart-fullness to identify specific names.

Yet I would like to acknowledge the heart of all the many brothers and sisters globally with whom I have sat in meditation. These experiences of unconditional love and silence are rare and precious. During my time as a student in India I experienced one of the most wonderful periods of learning and love in my life with Sravana, Vikram, Rakeesh

Acknowledgments

and Gayatri. Their heartfelt love and knowledge of Sanskrit and Yoga was delightful; their generosity in sharing with me life-changing. It was in their company that Yoga became a way of life and a way of being—not a class or an activity—something much more natural, integrated and relational. Although we are now separated by land and ocean, I often look at our last photo together and smile. I hope that this smile somehow crosses the distance between us and is felt as love

As always I offer all love and appreciation to my partner, my children, and whanau/family. The deep focus of writing requires a withdrawal in me from everyday activities, and I am grateful that this has been tolerated so kindly by my friends and loved ones. I would also like to acknowledge Heather Devere and Rhondda Davies for their editing, viewing, support and encouragement as the book took shape. And to Katerina Standish, what can I say? Without her passion, determination, and focus this book may have remained in gestation for much longer.

And finally I trust that those who find themselves reading this book will glimpse a deeper inner quietude. I view this book as a leaf that shelters a peaceful bud. You, the reader, are that potential peaceful flower. *Arohanui.*

Introduction

Yogic Peace Education seeks to transform. It goes beyond ordinary book learning towards the development of lived experience—towards transformation in those studying it and the communities in which they belong.

Education (of all kinds) is about learning. The aims of education are to provide the skills, knowledge, capability, morals, ethics, information and practices of life that individuals need to live and communities need to thrive. There is no "one size fits all" model of education; different students have different ways of learning just as different people exhibit different ways of thinking, being and believing. There are also many types of education and a multitude of ideas about what should and should not be included in education. Education can comprise accessing particular subjects, activities or ideas. Education can be a lifelong activity of autodidactic pursuits—one continues to learn as one continues to live and study and reflect and learn more. Education can be in institutional settings that one enters and exits after certain developmental stages or time periods. An education can pertain to a subject of study comprised of admittance (sometimes competitive or merit based), a liminal state of becoming *but not yet being* something (certifications or degrees that lead to professional work) or the mastery or completion of a specific area of exploration.

What education *encompasses* is the human transmission of cognitive, affective and behavioral ideals, values and norms. What education *does* is contribute to how we think, what we think about, how we feel and how we act. There is no question that what we learn can supply us with information that we absorb, consider, challenge, resist, champion and embody. But there is something *more* that education should teach us—show us, model for us and present as meaningful: self-knowledge. Yogic Science considers that knowledge has two forms—*jnana* and *vidya*. *Jnana* knowledge refers to knowledge that we gain through books, teachers and outside sources (intellectual knowledge) whereas *vidya* knowledge is the knowledge gained through intuitive and relational experience (wisdom). If education seeks to often (but not always) counter ignorance, the present work seeks to encourage our inner awareness; as a platform for learning to learn, live and love without violence—deliberate and avoidable harm. Yogic peace practitioners learn to master their own thought fields, developing a mind that is no longer susceptible to swings of emotion and misery. Such a mind is slow to react and learns the nuanced art of responsiveness. It is in such a mind that violence ceases to be an automatic reaction to pain or slights leaving it an entirely *negligible option*. What is encouraging is that such a mind can be developed regardless of culture, age, gender or stage.

We reiterate that violence is optional. Violence is deliberate harm or threat of harm; it is an event, a system, a worldview; incarnations of suffering, injury, destruction and dehumanization. But it is not the only option. The tools and techniques that follow will give teachers and learners the vital tools they need to cultivate a garden that is not only filled with *learnings* from the outside world but with the critical tools to foster self-knowledge, self-awareness and self-consciousness. This book recognizes that student/participants and teacher/facilitators appreciate that learning is not simply a cognitive procedure of acquiring information (Freire 2003) but a discipline of living that can shape the mind, affect the body, and touch the spirit. Noddings proclaims that what is needed in education is not more information of things external to the student regardless of their merits but "greater emphasis on self-knowledge" (2012, 80). This book seeks to supplement this assertion with valuable praxis that puts the work of gaining *self-knowledge* into learning space. As Synott reminds us, an "important feature of peace education and knowledge is its emphasis on praxis—the dialectic between theory and practice," and to this end this theory and practice manual aims to stimulate valuable peace praxis for peace practitioners (2006, 11).

As we move into the first decades of the 21st century, it serves us well, as a planet of bodies, shapes and systems, to move away from the extreme and at times systematic violence of the past (imperial ecology, colonialism, genocide, violence against women and children) to partner with one another in *nonviolence*—a principle of life that eschews harm done to others. Moreover, peace education is aligned with the interdisciplinary field of Peace and Conflict Studies—which emerged from Peace Studies and the study of interpersonal, intergroup and/or international conflict—but peace education is a tool that can also combat violence in the self. In a world where the leading cause of violent death worldwide is not terrorism or war or political or social revolution, but suicide—the act of killing oneself—a vital aperture of remedial necessity is more than called for.

Yogic Peace Education is more than a halcyon cry for a mindful turning away from violence but a deliberate antidote to violence of the self, violence done to others and violence in society. If the biggest task of peace education is "teaching people to listen to one another" (Noddings 2012, 141), the biggest task of yogic peace education is teaching people to *listen to themselves*. Once this happens it becomes natural to have the capability to listen to each other.

The following work will not only inform readers about how the disciplines of peace education and Yoga connect but will also provide useful and immediate practices of peace that teacher/learners can add to our educational tool kits. These techniques are thousands of years old but can only really be understood and appreciated through practice. Where so much of education is *learning about something*, yogic peace education is about a practical experience of peace and learning to communicate and act from that space. Yogic Peace Education is praxis for gaining self-knowledge that can be used in any educational setting. Yogic Peace Education is a way of teaching and learning that says there is a deep connection between self-realization and violence in the self and society, and there are manifold linkages between practicing nonviolence and building positive peace.

Peace education teaches us to recognize violence and act nonviolently; it teaches us that violence is not only an action but also part of our schools, societies and how we think. Peace education teaches us that living nonviolently is possible. Yogic peace education encourages us to take a step further by teaching us how to embody peace and learn to live and love in ways, which are responsive and inherently harmonious.

Introduction

It represents a human experience and manifestation of consciousness that celebrates unity within diversity and the development of human sensitivity that makes "heart-full" engagements natural. This book shares the ways in which this can become practical within the classroom, amongst peace practitioners and as an essential toolkit of those interested in the personal, community and planetary possibilities for peace.

PART I

PEACE EDUCATION

ONE

What Is Peace Education?

Introduction

Most explorations in the field of peace education begin with a thoughtful and considered delineation of what constitutes *peace* and what is meant by *peace education*. While this book will explore these terms in detail in subsequent pages it embraces Allen's (2007) outlook that the "goal of education [is] liberation: providing a means for service to meet the needs of others, for liberation from all forms of servitude and domination, and for one's ethical and spiritual liberation" (294). So what is peace education?

Peace education is a method of organized learning that contains principles and practices that aim to reduce or prevent violence and contribute to peace (Harris and Morrison 2013). The phrase "peace education" is associated with many different kinds of programs and can include educative offerings that incorporates broad and, at times vastly divergent, learning platforms. Peace education is values and attitudes, behaviors and mindsets. But, because peace education includes extensive and diverse learning agendas (not all programs cover identical material, include similar participants, are for the same duration; and not all teacher/facilitators hold matching qualifications), there has been significant critique and controversy (Salomon and Nevo 1999) of what is or is not peace education and whether the statement holds that because peace education can contain "everything" that it is, in fact, "nothing."

A multiplicity of meanings conveys the breadth of peace education. In some instances, peace education is *teaching for peace* (an objective)—

to reduce violence or increase social justice in society. In other examples, peace education relates to *teaching about peace*—learning about the subject of peace or processes that engage with pro-social elements such as democracy, conflict resolution and peaceful coexistence, including techniques used in conflict transformation such as negotiation or dialogue. Still other conceptualizations connect how this education is conducted—*teaching by peace*—using peace pedagogy or teaching styles that uphold the standards and aims of educating *for, by* and *about* peace and recognizing that education systems can be sites of violence, too.

What most definitions of peace education share—and for that matter programs that link the social process of education to building peace—is a meaningful association between learning, violence and alternatives to violence. Simply put, peace education helps us recognize violence—all types of violence; it considers violence destructive and considers the use of violence (even in response to violence) unacceptable. Further to this, peace education considers that we are individuals who "learn" violence; that many of us think that violence is "normal," and that it is possible to destabilize the common conclusion that humans are, have been, and will always be, violent (Fry 2007). It leads from this that peace education seeks to discover, analyze, understand and inevitably share tools and techniques that provide alternatives to violence (nonviolence or nonviolent methods) and, in doing so, to increase pro-social (and nonviolent) qualities and aptitudes that relate to a wide variety of human objectives including (but not limited to) social equality and justice, harmonious ecology, authentic and constructive relativity, and the eradication of suffering.

This book is a theory and practice manual for understanding and practicing Yogic Peace Education; it explores and articulates the connections between peace education and Yogic Science and then provides peace practitioners (in either classroom or community settings) with valuable tools and techniques for utilizing Yogic Peace Education. The goal of this volume is to firmly ground the yogic peace educator in the empirical and theoretical underpinnings of the discipline. As Harris comments, "peace educators cannot eliminate conflict but hey can provide students with valuable skills in managing conflict" (2004, 6) and to this end the purpose of this book is to both establish and then exercise the essential art of self-regulation. Chapter One begins by exploring

One. What Is Peace Education?

peace education and examining peace, conflict, violence and nonviolence. It then proceeds to identify and encapsulate typologies of peace education and types of peace educators.

Chapter Two introduces the theoretical construct of Johan Galtung's violence triangle and examines the hypothesis that direct, indirect (structural) and cultural forms of violence are linked, that they reinforce one another and that most forms of direct and indirect violence stem from social legitimizers found in cultural violence. This chapter inverts Galtung's configuration to argue that if cultural violence (as an aspect of culture) leads to direct and indirect violence then cultural *nonviolence* (as an aspect of culture) leads to direct and indirect nonviolence. If we can say facets of a culture are violent then peace education as a facet of culture that is nonviolent is a form of cultural *nonviolence*.

Chapter Three introduces yogic discipline and identifies the classical yogic pathways including *Raja, Hatha, Bhakti, Jnana* and *Karma Yoga*. This chapter relates the challenge of utilizing metaphysical concepts of Yoga in the modern era and offers a range of practices useful in preparing physiological systems for the experience of awareness and first-hand knowledge of our inherent union and connectivity (Yoga means to yoke or join). This chapter presents the Yoga psychology and philosophy behind Yogic Science and makes the suggestion that our perceptions of separateness from one another are a root of conflict that yogic practice can help to overcome.

Chapter Four is a scientific exploration of a core tenet of yogic practice: *ahimsa*. This practice (translated as non-harming, non-hurting or nonviolence) frequently considers and defines our actions to others (and what we do not do) but is rarely understood as a vehicle for eradicating personal violence. As Yoga describes practices that lead our neuropsychobiological systems towards balance, we ourselves become instruments of creative change. Peacebuilding, generally speaking, is an intervention and action that can lead to change. This chapter avers that Yogic Peace Education is a form of Yogic peacebuilding that stems from life-nourishing and life-cherishing values.

Chapter Five considers the value of practicing yogic peacebuilding as a group activity by investigating the idea of appropriate practice, alternative modalities within yoga and the premise that yoga is a practice (or range of practices) rather than an ideology. This chapter then considers the utility of yogic practices in particular groups of individuals including custodial and vulnerable populations and makes a proposition for the utilization of Yogic Peace Education in post-conflict communities.

Chapter Six presents the practice manual of this volume and how we learn to be instruments of wellness and peace. It sets out the five principles of Yogic Peace Education and then presents ten preparatory exercises. The chapter then introduces three toolkits that the yogic peace educator can utilize in appropriate settings: learning without violence; living without violence; and loving without violence. It concludes by reiterating a primary goal of the book: it should stand as a manual of self-investigation that can be shared.

Defining Peace, Conflict, Violence and Nonviolence

WHAT IS PEACE?

When a concept is defined it furthers a shared sense of understanding. When something is a concrete substance—like wood, for instance—it is relatively simple to define (wood is a fibrous material derived from trees); in other circumstances, defining something with abstract qualities—such as the concept of peace—is more challenging. There are perceptions that peace refers to all things positive, "a master concept" that includes aspired-to and actual ways-of-being and behaving (Bar-Tal 2002, 27). As the concept of peace has both tangible and intangible qualities, peace can be (and is) conceived of, in many different ways.

Common descriptions of peace include:

- Absence of war
- Lack of interpersonal disagreement
- Freedom from hostility
- Tranquility, serenity or calmness

Peace scholars and students use additional terms to differentiate types of peace, including:

- Negative peace (absence of direct violence) (Galtung 1996)
- Positive peace (absence of structural violence) (Galtung 1996)
- Sustainable peace (prevention of conflict) (Lederach 1995)
- Stable peace (low probability of war) (Boulding 1978)
- Perpetual peace (permanent negative peace) (Kant 1983)
- Just peace (economic justice) (Annan 2005)
- World peace (a conflict-free globe) (Walker 1988)

There are terms that refer to specific undertakings or actions that relate to peace, such as:

- Peacekeeping (military maintenance of negative peace)
- Peacemaking (creating peace agreements between conflict parties)
- Peacebuilding (interventions that increase peace and inhibit violence)
- Pacifism (rejection of war, refusal to contribute to war)

Finally, there are more esoteric conceptualizations of peace that include states of being that relate to practice and discipline such as:

- Inner peace
- Being at peace
- Peace of mind
- Making peace with something
- Enlightenment
- Positive consciousness

The cultural roots of peace are vast, varied and ever changing. Peace was once a term that indicated an end to war but now the word peace is aligned with many aims, objectives and conditions that are more meaningful and range far wider. How one defines peace is relative to how one conceives of peace, how one contributes to peace and how one imagines peace to be.

What Is Conflict?

Conflict according to the *Oxford English Dictionary* (2016) is discord—a struggle, opposition, disagreement, resistance, differing opinions or an outright dispute. And although violence can emerge from conflict not all forms of conflict are violent. Conflict relates to identity, resources, goals and one's perspective (Burton 1990; Lederach 2005; Volkan 2006). Conflict generally appears in the individual when there is unease of some kind, a feeling that something is not quite right. Conflict occurs between individuals or groups when two or more (individuals or groups) occupy the same space and their proximity leads either to a competition for goods, prestige or power or to the amplification of different and seemingly incompatible, opinions, beliefs or feelings. Conflict emerges between cultural groups (religious, national or ethnic groups, or identity groups united by other qualities) when discord is rooted in how people are treated, how they see themselves and how they see one another.

Although conflict is often depicted as a negative form of rivalry, competition or enmity, conflict can be productive, creative (Boulding 2000) or an act that is positively conflictual (Mouffe 1995). Without conflict there is no metamorphosis, no growth and no transformation (Lederach 2005). While some conflict is destructive and oppressive, other conflicts lead to positive changes, and affirming and pro-social amendments—for example, the advent of the United Nations (UN) Universal Declaration of Human Rights (1948). Subsequent conventions, such the Convention on the Elimination of all forms of Discrimination against Women (1979), the UN Declaration of the Rights of the Child (1989) or the Convention on the Rights of Persons with Disabilities (2006) are the result of continued conflicts and address discords not reflected in the foundational human rights document (Donnelly 2013). Conflict is a part of life and it requires attention, investigation, consideration and engagement. Conflict left unexamined can lead to greater discord. Conflict disregarded can lead to violence.

What Is Violence?

Violence is an unfortunate part of the human world. Violence can be part of a system (structural violence), an action (direct violence) or part of a worldview (cultural violence) but all violence involves inflicting harm (or threatening harm) and causing suffering (Galtung 1990). And with the aim of gaining a foothold in understanding what violence is, it is critical to understand that forms of violence often follow a trajectory of influence. Many acts of violence are perceived as "one-offs" or singular events that are independent acts of aggression between distinct individuals. Galtung's theory of Cultural Violence (1990), however, posits that all forms of violence have cultural origins and that, when one is trying to fathom the complexity of violence, it is necessary to understand that the roots of structural violence (institutionalized, invisible) and direct violence (agentic, visible) lie in cultural violence. Cultural violence includes symbolic aspects of cultures that make structural and direct forms of violence legitimate—and make them "look, even feel, right—or at least not wrong" (Galtung 1990, 291.) This leads to the conclusion that compartmentalizing violence can act to recognize acts of harm but that acts of harm are not isolated from cultural aspects that in some way, shape or form make using violence permissible.

Defining violence is a complex and complicated endeavor. Violence can be divided into specific incarnations (for example, physical abuse, sexual abuse, financial abuse and psychological abuse); it can be separated into types of violence (personal, interpersonal, social, cyber); it can include medical categories (post-traumatic, antisocial, psychopathic or sociopathic violence); or it can be classified according to victims; those in turn sub-classified as vulnerable populations, e.g., women and children (Englander 2007).

There are many official definitions of violence, including:

- Behavior involving physical force intended to hurt, damage, or kill someone or something (OED).
- The intentional use of physical force or power, threatened or actual, against oneself, another person, or against a group or community, which either results in or has a high likelihood of resulting in injury, death, psychological harm, maldevelopment, or deprivation (World Health Organization).
- An extreme form of aggression, such as assault, rape or murder (American Psychological Association).

Further to this, particular forms of violence have more targeted definitions such as the UN definition of violence against women (VAW):

- act of gender-based violence that results in, or is likely to result in, physical, sexual or psychological harm or suffering to women, including threats of such acts, coercion or arbitrary deprivation of liberty, whether occurring in public or in private life.

The UN definition of violence against children:

- all forms of physical or mental violence, injury and abuse, neglect or negligent treatment, maltreatment or exploitation, including sexual abuse.

Definitions of political violence commonly use these descriptions:

- acts of aggression that are motivated by a desire to gain or maintain political power including government repression, riots, coups, civil wars, insurgencies, crime rings, gendercide, ethnic cleansing or genocide (cultural or instrumental or both).

There are numerous typologies of violence. Violence can be separated into personal (self-directed), interpersonal, or collective:

1. Personal violence: self-harm or suicide.
2. Interpersonal violence: violence between two individuals.
   - Intimate violence—*this often takes place in the home*—violence between intimates (family members or partners), including elders or children.
   - Community violence—*this often takes place in public*—violence between unrelated, unacquainted people or strangers.
3. Collective violence: violence perpetrated by groups such as states, political groups or insurgent groups.

The term abuse is frequently considered to mean the same thing as violence. The term abuse is similar but marginally distinct—abuse normally refers to mistreatment and is often (but not always) between persons who are not equals). Types of abuse can contain:

- Physical abuse: when someone physically harms another person.
- Sexual abuse: when a person is sexualized, sexually humiliated or unwillingly made to participate in sexual activities.
- Financial abuse: when someone controls (or takes without a person's consent) another's money or resources.

- Neglect: when someone is unwilling and fails to care for someone they are responsible for.
- Emotional abuse: humiliation or harmful actions that make a person lose dignity and wellbeing.
- Psychological abuse: manipulation or threats of harm that cause fear and mental suffering.
- Cultural abuse: when a person's cultural beliefs permit or require them to harm someone else.
- Verbal and literary abuse: when someone uses words, either spoken or written, in person or online, to hurt another individual.

Violence can be categorized by its social or cultural regard—what is tolerated or acceptable in any social or cultural group—and divided into, for example, legitimate (self-defense, punishment, the military) or illegitimate (interpersonal harm, belligerence, militancy) forms (Felson 2009). Legitimate forms of violence are culturally contingent—what is considered acceptable and what is culturally condoned vary depending on your cultural position, your cultural beliefs, personal opinions and the amount of power you hold in your relative social group.

What Is Nonviolence?

Nonviolence is a term that encompasses a number of political, practical and philosophical positions and can include action, inaction, a stratagem, a mental discipline or a worldview (Kurlansky 2006). Although the word nonviolence seems to indicate a passive "not doing," in actual fact nonviolence is a vibrant, active and robust force of wellbeing and love. The following section will briefly examine three common forms of nonviolence: pacifism, principled nonviolence and pragmatic nonviolence.

Pacifism

Pacifism is a term that encompasses a variety of ideological positions (minimal, contingent, absolute, maximal, and universal) but is most usually associated with the custom of opposing war, military aggression and the use of physical force (Brock and Young 1999). A pacifist may choose to abstain from using force to achieve any number of objectives on either moral or practical grounds ("it is wrong" and/or "it won't work"). And pacifism, as a modern "peace" practice, follows a custom of nonviolence that is found historically and geographically all over the world.

The Jains, Buddhists and Mohists of South Asia, the Moriori of the South Pacific, and the early Christians and Bogomils of Europe all practiced nonviolence (Gier 2004). By the 17th century, the Christian Peace Churches (Church of the Brethren, Quakers, Amish, Mennonites, and Hutterites) refused to obey laws of military conscription and perform any actions of outward aggression. This refusal was based on the moral values of nonviolence espoused by Jesus in the New Testament (Trocmé 1961).

Pacifist ideals in the Western world are closely associated with Christianity (Merton 1980) and the historical opposition to several forms of international aggression, most notably the Napoleonic wars, the Crimean war and World War I (Roth 2002). For modern pacifists, war is an unacceptable undertaking regardless of the outcome. Pacifist acts can include refusing to do military service or contribute to state apparatuses that support war (taxes), instead pursuing other acts that revere life, including vegetarianism, opposing the death penalty, euthanasia and medical termination of pregnancy (McCarthy 2002).

A leading spiritual prophet of pacifism and nonviolence was undoubtedly Leo Tolstoy, whose 1894 work *The Kingdom of God is Within You* served as inspiration to these later proponents of nonviolence, civil resistance and social revolution—Mohandas K. Gandhi, Bertha von Suttner and Martin Luther King, Jr. While Tolstoy was a devout follower of Jesus of Nazareth, he firmly believed that resistance to the doctrines of Christianity (the powerful Christian Orthodox Church of Russia) was essential because they contradicted Christ's commandment of "non-resistance to evil by force," (Jesus' Sermon on the Mount commanded that one do good to those who would harm one and surrender to one's enemies, famously "turning the other cheek" when faced with aggression). This sentiment is legendarily echoed in the words of Christian monk, Thomas Merton, who wrote that nonviolence demands "that one be ready to suffer evil and even face the threat of death without violent retaliation ... [and that] Christian nonviolence is not built on a presupposed division, but on the *basic unity of man*"(emphasis added) (Merton 1980, 208–9).

Christian theologian Saint Augustine of Hippo's doctrine of a "just war" (where war is considered a moral method to bring about peace if certain conditions are met) (Shaw 2003), can here be contrasted with Tolstoy's tenet that war is never just and that church sanctioned war is both abhorrent and unconditionally incompatible with true belief in Christ's teachings.

Christian pacifists do not place membership (for example, national citizenship) of any human organization above their allegiance to the laws of God as communicated by Jesus Christ. Similar to the notion of total Islam (the Islamic religion is a totality that encompasses all spheres of living and does not distinguish between political and spiritual life) (Armstrong, 2005) to Christian pacifists, also, the state is subordinate to God and it can neither force compliance (through, for instance, military conscription) nor provide spiritual salvation. This is spiritually echoed in Henry Thoreau's 1849 maxim that humans—male ones at the time—should be "men first and subjects second."

PRINCIPLED NONVIOLENCE AND *AHIMSA*

The field of nonviolence is not effortlessly comprehended, as there are a variety of practices, traditions, actions and intentions along the nonviolence spectrum. Some pacifists espouse values that are synonymous with principled nonviolence and some groups, who utilize pragmatic strategies of nonviolent defense, have principled intentions (Burrowes 1996). What can be said is that Western (Christian) pacifism has echoes of the Eastern practice of *ahimsa*—a non-harming virtue of the highest order.

The Eastern virtue of non-harming (a form of principled nonviolence) is also interpreted to mean "being nonviolent" or not causing pain. *Ahimsa*, as it was originally conceived, was a Hindu practice for individual perfection and was a prescribed practice for spiritual professionals (monks, priests, renunciates). *Ahimsa* is aligned with the mental discipline of the interrogation of the ego, the cultivation of truth or truth awareness and the rejection of violence. A dedicated Buddhist, for instance, considers negative emotions and violent behaviors the result of attachment to material goods (or people) and utilizes mental disciplines of non-attachment to change personal human conduct. A *yogin* (follower of Yogic Science) acts in ways to minimize harmful behaviors and attitudes to decrease the destructive effects of violence on the human instrument. *Ahimsa*, the discipline of non-harming, is considered a foundational discipline in many spiritual practices and teaches that violence is not only *never the right option* but is *a totally destructive exploit* that affects both the agent(s) and the victim(s) of violence.

Gandhian *Ahimsa*

In the modern age, Gandhian *ahimsa* is distinct from classical *ahimsa* in that it is a daily practice that can be of benefit to anybody not just spiritual specialists. Gandhian *ahimsa* combines the disciplines of non-harming (nonviolence, vegetarianism) with the directives of living with what the Greeks termed *agápe*—humanly love. For Gandhi *ahimsa* did not simply mean not doing something (restraining violence) but actively doing something else (executing love). Gandhian *ahimsa* encompasses the directive of doing the least amount of harm possible while giving the most amount of love imaginable. Gandhi termed this practice *satyagraha*—*satya* (truth) *graha* (force)—and he believed that when using this practice, we must begin by transforming our own inner violence before we can use compassion and patience to change the hearts of our opponents (Gandhi 1983). For Gandhi, violence was proof that we perceived of the "other" as separate from ourselves. If we perceive of the unity of all life, then violence is no longer an option. Gandhian *ahimsa* affirms the unity of all sentient beings and is both a restraint (from violence) and an observance (of love).

Pragmatic Nonviolence

Pragmatic Nonviolence refers to particular practices that are used to transform political structures. Pragmatic nonviolence includes utilizing nonviolent resistance (civil disobedience) in social movements as a "strategy" of nonviolent defense. Pragmatic nonviolence is utilized by dozens of revolutionary parties who, historically, might have chosen armed struggle to both dissent from, and transform, society (Sharp 2005). The strategy of nonviolent defense (pragmatic nonviolence) is based on the notion that true power does not rest in the hands of political functionaries (police, military or governments) but in the hands of individual people (the public). Pragmatic nonviolence aims to systematically destabilize the support structures of a society to affect political change. There are a number of qualities of nonviolent defense that make pragmatic nonviolence successful: it can include anyone, because it requires total restraint from using violence (even in defense of violence) it invites participation and because it does not use violence it allows its followers to uphold the moral high ground in the face of (frequent) violence repression (Sharp 2005). Studies have shown that nonviolent strategies work (much better than violent ones) and pragmatic nonviolence is an available option because individuals and groups can use it regardless of their ideological, spiritual or religious positions (Stephan and Chenoweth, 2008).

A Summary of Nonviolence

Pacifism is a refusal to participate in violence (especially state organized violence); pragmatic nonviolence is a strategic discipline that works to change society or obtain a political outcome, whereas principled nonviolence contains an internal dimension comprising an ethical restraint on expressions of any form of violence for any reason. Simply put, a principled nonviolence advocate never feels that violence is permissible and pragmatic nonviolence advocate feels that nonviolence is more successful when working toward social transformation. What all of these nonviolent traditions share is a sense that violence is an unacceptable action, even in response to violence. While some consider violence as it is usually defined, others include all acts that have the potential to cause harm.

Most famously, Gandhi and Dr. Martin Luther King Jr. successfully utilized nonviolent strategies during the quest for home rule in India and the civil rights struggle in the United States respectively, but nonviolent resistance has also been used elsewhere. Nonviolence was used in the Māori village of Parihaka (in contemporary New Zealand) to resist European colonial occupation in 1881; and it was a strategy of social transformation during various soft revolutions in several ex–Soviet bloc countries (for example, Czechoslovakia, Lithuania); it was used in Latin America (Brazil, Argentina); and also Asia (Thailand, the Philippines). The Global Nonviolence Index lists over 800 instances where nonviolent strategies were utilized and includes case studies from almost every country in the world. These traditions share an important moral and ethical platform with peace education. In peace education, violence is not acceptable.

> KATERINA: I teach courses in Peace and Conflict Studies and Peace Education in a university setting right now but I used to do far more community based education that gave me a broad appreciation of how "where" we learn/know affects "what" we learn/know. I used to teach and learn with students from all walks of life in Yoga studios, recreation facilities and community centers involving practices designed for scholarship, self-care and fitness and often focused around youth, mental illness, pregnancy, injury and lifestyle challenges that included substance abuse and self-harming. All of these experiences have shown me that how a person engages with concepts like, peace, conflict, violence and nonviolence are really affected by the setting in which one encounters such terms and such experiences. In academic settings people use "accepted" definitions, and are constantly concerned they don't correctly understand something whereas in community settings people always relate terms such as these to their lives: violence in their life, peace in their life, conflict in their life. The greatest gap that I see is an understanding that the majority of the time, in the numerous mundane and everyday settings people behave non-violently but totally without awareness of it. When you indicate that in their personal reportage they are acting nonviolently they are usually surprised that is a "thing." We, as a global species, spend all this time focusing on violence (responses to violence, prevention of violence, punishment of violence) and too little time thinking about peace or nonviolence. The norm is nonviolence, but we don't seem to see it that way. As one of my students said to me: "Nonviolence ... is that a thing?"

> JANINE: I was pondering the line "nonviolence—is that even a thing?" In fact I had a dream about it. In the dream I was reminded that from a Yogic science perspective the Self is pure and without attributes. In a sense not framed as violent or nonviolent—rather pure love and potentiality. From this base it is up to us what we want to accept or not accept in our lives. It is up to us what we choose to create in our minds and in our conditioning. What we allow to be reinforced. The current neoliberal ideas are just one way for the human mind to be conditioned. Its values encourage human suffering and violence as the inequality is unsustainable. Yet there are other values and ways of expressing ourselves as human beings. As I look at the suffering on the planet it seems that creating a human mind free of the neoliberal conditioning is a work for heroes and heroines. It will require the quiet inner work and outer actions of many of us.

Typologies of Peace Education

Peace education encompasses a variety of pro-peace (peace enhancing) platforms. Harris and Morrison (2013) divide peace education into five categories: human rights education, international education, development education, conflict resolution education and education for sustainability.

Freedom and Dignity: Human Rights Education

This form of peace education is a defense against injustice and is based on the idea that there are natural laws of humanity—independent of social, religious or political bodies—and these laws recognize that *every human being* possesses the rights enshrined in the Universal Declaration of Human Rights (and later documents). They champion inherent and inalienable human dignity and the right to freedom from abuse. Education, that works toward the awareness of injustice and the acquisition of multicultural values, coexistence practices, cultural consciousness and countering prejudice, can be considered education for human rights.

Peace and the Planet: Education for Sustainability

Sustainability refers to the relationship between humanity and the environment and either develops environmental consideration (caring for water systems or aiding endangered species) or the utilization of resources (managing consumption) to ensure our ability in the future to sustain life. In a way, education for sustainability places the human experience into an ecosystem, imparts knowledge and supports understanding our impact on the natural world. Education for sustainability shares and fosters attitudes and behaviors that support a future-minded consumption of natural resources and environmental stewardship.

The World System: International Education

Earth—the planet we all live on—is an increasingly interconnected and interdependent site of human activity. As discrete communities disappear, we come to appreciate that the world (as a result of the long and continuing process of globalization) is a matrix of increasingly connected systems of economics, technology, politics and culture. There are global systems that exist within individual states, work between states and work independent of states. There are cultural structures that transcend spatial origins and unifying constructs that seek to create platforms of international engagement and responsibility. International education seeks to explain how the world works, to examine the world beyond individual borders, understand the impact and effects of living in a globalized world and foster global citizenry. Included in international education is information about global structures such as the United Nations or the impact of global engagements such as the disarmament movements of the 20th century.

Learning Alternatives: Conflict Resolution Education

Learning to manage discord is a common concern for peace educators. Conflict resolution education involves learning platforms that provide an individual with the tools to assess conflict, communicate effectively, assess their relationships and create positive changes in their social world. This form of peace education is concerned with how we relate to one another and how to transform violent relationships. Conflict resolution education can involve courses that teach students to become aware of conflict and violence, deal with conflict nonviolently, manage conflict when they see it, prevent violence from happening and learn pro-social peacemaking behaviors that contribute to personal, interpersonal and community wellbeing.

Inclusive Economies: Development Education

Inequality and economic disparities are the results of multiple social and cultural processes over time that leads to violence. The goal of development education is to understand the connection between material resources and wellbeing, and to identify and destabilize dominance structures that further inequality. This form of peace education is both global and local and the nature of inquiry and remedy relate to the importance of meeting needs without taking resources that belong to other people, other species and future generations. Development education is concerned with social justice, critical consciousness and ethical resource allocation. Peace educators that teach development education share information about the economic systems that impact social reality and impart ways to increase local ownership and enjoyment of important resources.

An alternative conceptualization is offered by Haavelsrud (1996) who considers there to be four attitudes or "approaches" to peace education programming including the idealist approach; intellectual approach; ideological approach; and politicization approach. In this typology peace education offerings fit into categories with distinct philosophies or ideals. The *idealist approach* in peace education is concerned with notions of universal truth, "what should be," and this approach pays little attention to structural realities on the ground, focusing instead on mindsets and new ways of thinking. An *intellectual approach* to peace education seeks to generate scholarly and scientific "peace findings" that can be accessed by interested parties. The intellectual approach is described as being more concerned with generating "peace data" than with affecting social/cultural change. The *ideological approach* considers all schooling to be an instrument of social control and maintains the necessity that peace education offerings be accessible only "outside" mainstream education. This approach maintains that in order to be effective peace education programs must remain on the margins of contemporary education. The final tactic, the *politicization approach*, encompasses peace education programs that are committed to social change "in schools" as a part of greater society. This approach sees the need to critically engage students as change agents in society and considers education systems as suitable loci for building peace.

Bajaj (2008) adds the *critical peace education approach* which sees the purpose of peace education as supporting the development of critical consciousness (Freire 2003) and a deep and critical *rooting* of peace education in an understanding of local realities including culture, identity and access to power. In this conceptualization of critical peace education, peace educators are cautioned to recognize the potential of their "educations" to destabilize learners when established (normally Western) notions of building peace either ignore local peace potentialities or transplant culturally incongruous dogma into places where Western values and resident social reality are quite dissimilar (Snauwaert 2011).

Where Bajaj champions a critical peace education approach that connects the act of learning/teaching to global structural inequality and social justice, Standish (2015) considers critical peace education as a pedagogical strategy to embrace inclusivity. Critical peace education in this view must not only investigate, recognize or understand inequality but the "practice of critical pedagogy in peace education requires that ... when critical pedagogues are educating for peace they are not simply looking for those who have, and those who *have less* (or at least are perceived so) but are looking to create radical love in the classroom" (Standish 2015, 32). This critical peace education approach begins the action of social transformation with individuals—to not only support practices of critical consciousness but also "destabilize identity characteristics and reveal inherent human dignity" (Standish 2015, 32). In addition to the aforementioned types of peace education, there are *coexistence educations* (educations that seek to create bonds between parties in discord), *dialogue educations* (educations that teach communication tools for speaking without violence) or *violence reduction educations* (educations that address certain forms of social violence and its reduction/cessation). Although a student of peace education learns to appreciate the many platforms of understanding available in a peace education tool kit there is still an additional quality of peace education regarding not merely *what* is taught but *why* and *how* it is taught. Building upon many of the pre-existing typologies surveyed in this chapter, the next section will posit that not only are there different kinds of peace education, *there are different kinds of peace educators* and offers an elementary classification of peace educators into Montessorian, Galtungian, Reardonian, Freireian and Ghandian (see Table 1).

Types of Peace Educators

This section seeks to inquire of peace educators: what type of peace educator are you? It speaks to the emphasis, orientation and active offerings of five innovative peace educators and explores their focus, locus and toolkit. The five types are presented here as platforms for engaging with education as a tool for building peace. Should the reader be interested there are ample sources from which to gain particular depths of understanding from the biographies and pracademic (practitioner-academic) discourses that emerge from each educator surveyed here and, in addition to these five types, many more outlooks, practices and positions to contemplate. In this next section attention will not be placed on what peace educators hold in common but rather, what makes each peace educator *different*.

Montessorian

Focus
Child Development: inclusive, autonomous, child-led learning with teacher as director/observer—education offerings that instill in children the qualities of self-motivation, self-reliance, self-discipline.

Locus
School: classrooms and outside places as spaces of liberation where children can individually and spontaneously develop emotionally, mentally, morally and physically. Peace through pedagogical transformation.

Toolkit
Care-based activities: teaching children to be responsible for themselves, the environment and for others with practices that include hygiene and wellness activities such as food preparation and physical fitness.

Galtungian

Focus
Knowledge: awareness of the multiplicities of violence present in society (direct, indirect and cultural), the interconnectivity of violence(s), the genesis/trajectory of violence(s) and the necessity of positive (sustainable) peacebuilding.

Locus
Academic-research centers: social institutions as spaces of recognition and awareness—comprehensive deliberation that leads to social/cultural nonviolence. Peace through cognitive transformation.

Toolkit

Critical inquiry: interdisciplinary empirical and theoretical inquiry that unearths visible and invisible social/cultural mechanisms of oppression and dehumanization.

REARDONIAN

Focus

Equality-Unity: Human Rights, Global Citizenship Education, Earth (planetary) Interconnectivity.

Locus

Schools: primary, secondary and tertiary educational spaces as places where social value systems are recognized and generated. Peace through planetary transformation.

Toolkit

Intentional education: cooperative education, global peace learning, noncompetition training, Military/Sexism nexus awareness and War System recognition, nonviolent crisis consciousness and the delegitimization of gender binaries.

FREIREIAN

Focus

Liberation: social/political transformation of adults through emancipatory education and critical pedagogy—cognizance of education systems as vehicles for domination and the opportunities through education for personal and social freedom.

Locus

Communities: individual education as an avenue toward full humanity. Peace through community transformation.

Toolkit

Critical consciousness: action-reflection (Praxis) consciousness, participatory learning, community education, literacy training.

Ghandian

Focus
Personal alteration: individual training and personal discipline that lead to (first) a moral-cultural character shift and (afterward) interpersonal concurrence and universal peace.

Locus
Individual: peace through individual transformation.

Toolkit
Spiritual-ethical-moral education: means-ends interconnectivity awareness, personal observance-restraint training, physical purity practice (including nutrition, physical fitness and contemplative practices).

TABLE 1
Five Types of Peace Educators

	Focus	Locus	Toolkit	
Montessorian	Child Development	Early Childhood-Primary	Care Activities	Peace through Pedagogical Transformation
Galtungian	Knowledge	Academic-research centres	Critical inquiry	Peace through Cognitive Transformation
Reardonian	Equality-Unity	Primary-Secondary-Tertiary	Intentional education	Peace through Planetary Transformation
Freireian	Liberation	Communities	Critical consciousness	Peace through Community Transformation
Ghandian	Personal transformation	Individual	Spiritual-ethical-moral education	Peace through Individual Transformation

Conclusions

Understanding nuances of peace, conflict, violence and nonviolence is one aim of peace education. As peace education is concerned with recognizing and reducing (or eliminating) violence in society and fostering positive peace, there is merit in considering how such terms are perceived, conceived and employed. The main "takeaway" from this exploration of the concepts of peace, conflict, violence and nonviolence, relates to the important understanding that a conflict left unexamined can lead to more discord and, in some instances, a conflict ignored can lead to violence. Awareness of our world, our actions and our mindsets is often a foundation of a peace education offering and the purpose is not only to expose and investigate *how* we make the world but also to understand that there are *other ways* the world can be made.

There are many different kinds of education(s) found in a peace education toolkit. Some relate to emphasis (human rights, sustainability, internationalism, development or interpersonal communication), orientation (idealist, intellectual, ideological or politicization) or objective (alternative education, liberation, personal or planetary peace) but each form and focus in peace education is based upon a recognition that whereas conflict is a normal (even desirable) facet of humanity, violence—deliberate harm done to others—is neither normal nor desirable and, in fact, is essentially utterly avoidable.

Cultural violence includes facets of culture that in some way legitimize direct (physical) or indirect (structural) forms of violence. Cultural nonviolence includes facets of culture that in some way *delegitimize* direct or indirect violence (Standish 2014). In the next chapter we examine peace education as a form of cultural nonviolence.

TWO

Peace Education as Cultural Nonviolence

Introduction[1]

There is a foundational tenet in peace education which pronounces that violence should never be employed in response to a conflict. Nonviolence (non-aggression, non-harming, non-hurting, non-killing), deeply rooted in many different cultures can been seen as a close sibling to modern peacebuilding. Such roots extend significantly into the role of education in conflict, learning and peace as education systems generate and reflect cultural values. Past, present and future peace educators will adhere, to greater or lesser degrees, to this tenet depending upon how they imagine violence but it cannot be ignored that the cultural roots of nonviolence since the twentieth century, that relate to ideological pursuits and issues of societal and social change, consider violence (in at least some form) as an illegitimate and/or undesirable act (Stephan and Chenoweth 2008; Clements 2008).

The United Nations Educational, Scientific and Cultural Organization (UNESCO) avers that "in the new turbulent international globalized landscape … greater account must be taken of the close links between cultural diversity, dialogue, development, security and peace" (2013, 2). While this statement could motivate a person to optimistically encounter difference, engage with others, and work together toward a safe and sustainable existence—all activities that contribute to positive peace—it does not emerge from any specific cultural standpoint and perhaps suggests that by appreciating, for example, cultural diversity, positives outcomes will appear. These two objectives are part of the conceptual backdrop of positive peace: "the presence of symbiosis and equity in human relations" (Galtung 1996, 14); and the perception that peace is not merely the absence of direct violence but the absence of structural (discrimination, marginalization, inequality) violence too.

Culture is a shared, socially transmitted system of meaning that has both physical and symbolic forms (Ross 2007). Culture can refer to the language a person speaks, their religious practices, but also other, less obvious, forms of social life such as schooling, science or art. For peace educators, the connection between culture and learning has already been made recognizing the great impact that socialization (primary and secondary) have on the transmission of cultural values, attitudes and behaviors. This is impacted by the growing connectivity in our communities where, in our "increasingly globalized landscape" (UNESCO, 2013, 2), we are in constant contact with *otherness*—ways of living, perceiving and believing that differ from our own, and that broaden and challenge our cultural landscape.

There are a variety of perspectives concerning cultural diversity and peace. While some imagine a space of destructive intercultural encounter (Huntington 1996), others imagine that appropriate exposure to even more others leads to a decrease in prejudice and an increase in positive regard (Allport 1954; Pettigrew 1998). More recent scholars grapple with evidence that when we encounter people from other cultures and the experience is negative, we tend to ascribe negative characteristics to the whole group (Paolini, Harwood and Rubin 2010).

In terms of violence, Galtung (1990) reminds us that all forms of violence—whether direct or structural in nature—have cultural roots. Direct violence includes acts or threats of aggression or harm that trespass on the integrity of the human instrument (the somatic and mental body). Discrimination and prejudice are forms of structural violence, social structures that deny individuals and groups the ability to satisfy human needs such as survival, well-being, recognition and freedom (Galtung 1996, 1990).

Encounters with *otherness* have led to some spectacularly destructive results such as female subordination, slavery, the devastation of the natural world and the subjugation of indigenous populations through colonization. However, the increasingly globalized world and the encounter of other cultures can also be seen (optimistically) as increasing the human potential for peace by sharing ways of seeing, being and behaving. These ways are based on celebrating and manifesting peaceabilities for the betterment of all living things. The following section investigates whether or not the theoretical construct of cultural violence (the root of all other forms of violence) has a functional opposite—*cultural nonviolence*—and then declares the discipline of peace education to be a form of cultural nonviolence. In the next section, cultural violence will be defined, two incarnations of non-harming will be examined—Gandhian *ahimsa* and pragmatic nonviolence—and peace education will be investigated as a form of cultural nonviolence.

Cultural Violence

Johan Galtung developed the construct of cultural violence to explain how direct (threatening) and structural (indirect) forms of violence are legitimized in society (1990). In his article, *Violence, Peace and Peace Research* published in 1969, Galtung explored perceptible and imperceptible forms of violence in society to make visible the reality that discrimination, inequality and prejudice are just as harmful and destructive as physical acts of violence (or threats of the same) but that they are distinguished from acts of direct violence because they cannot be tied to a specific agent. *Cultural Violence* (1990) built upon Galtung's prior theorizing to include the symbolic spheres of life and discovered that it is within such symbolic spheres that the roots of direct and indirect violence lie. Importantly for this volume, included in such a symbolic sphere is the act of educating.

Cultural violence refers to "'aspects of cultures,' not entire cultures [because] entire cultures can hardly be classified as violent" (Galtung 1990, 291). Cultural violence exists in the symbolic sphere of life "exemplified by religion and ideology, language and art, empirical science and formal science ... stars, crosses and crescents; flags, anthems and military parades; the ubiquitous portrait of the Leader; inflammatory speeches and posters" and other symbolic forms that hold social meaning such as schooling (Galtung 1990, 291). Cultural violence is important because it makes direct and structural violence "look, even feel, right—or at least not wrong" (Galtung 1990, 291). Cultural violence is important because without it other forms of violence would not be tolerated in society.

Gandhian Ahimsa

As explored elsewhere in this manuscript, the Sanskrit word *ahimsa* can be translated as non-harming, or not-hurting. The word is attributed to the Indian sage Patanjali, who listed it first among his universal ethics of personal transformation in the eight-limbed (*Ashtanga*) path. The *Yoga Sutras* affirm that "when [the *yogin*] is grounded in [the virtue of] nonharming (*ahimsâ*), enmity ceases in his presence (2.35)" (Feuerstein 2001, 224). The observance (*yama*) of *ahimsa*, or discipline of non-harming (nonviolence), appears in the Buddhist noble eightfold path, the Jain *Agamas* and later teachings of monotheistic human spirituality.

Yoga, emerging over thousands of years of study and practice, can be considered a Hindu psychotechnology for personal perfection (Feuerstein 2001). As all life was considered sacred to ancient Indian sages, the act of destroying life was considered highly problematic. *Ahimsa* has classically been associated with renunciates, such as monks, people who leave daily living behind for a life of spiritual pursuit. However, even to the renunciate, *ahimsa* did not entail the total absence of violence as it was recognized that "to live was to kill ... [as] every living being lived on some other living being" (Parehk 1988, 195). For *yogins*, Buddhist monks or Jain monks, the total avoidance of harming other life was considered impossible so the observation of *ahimsa* entailed minimizing violence and whenever possible abstaining from acts of destruction.

Mohandas K. Gandhi was a modern political and cultural thinker who was deeply influenced by Indian spirituality and world religion. While the scope of this work does not permit an exhaustive exploration of the life and pursuits of Gandhi (there are hundreds of volumes more suited to this purpose should the reader desire to do so), Gandhi's perception (some would term, re-conception) of *ahimsa* is a valuable point from which to examine "living" *ahimsa*, a form of *nonviolence* that begins with personal transformation.

Whereas *ahimsa* was originally a methodology employed to move toward personal spiritual perfection (renunciates practice monastic discipline in order to experience divinity—the interconnectivity of all existence), to Gandhi the discipline of *ahimsa* required "broadening" to "suit the needs of the age" (Parekh 1988, 200). Gandhi conceived of *ahimsa* as a custom that held the positive practice of non-harming intact but added a facet of love "both passive and active love, refraining from causing harm and destruction to living beings and positively promoting their well-being" (Parekh 1988, 200). Gandhi included love within his conceptualization of *ahimsa* not only to identify with the importance of acting non-harmfully but also to include in the undertaking the provision of life nourishing amenities to others. Gandhian *ahimsa* was both restraint and observation—doing minimal harm while giving love.

Gandhi experienced both direct and indirect violence in South Africa and India in the first half of the 20th century. Afterward, Gandhi became convinced that the use of violence to overcome violence would never result in peace, "violence ... maximizes ontological separateness and divisiveness and is based on the fundamental belief that the other ... is essentially different from me or us" (Allen 2007, 302). Gandhi believed that the primary struggle against violence happened "within" an individual and that it was the illusion of separateness (our separateness from each other) that led people to differentiate, judge or condemn one another. Gandhi envisioned violence as more than the destruction of living beings; he saw it as an affront to unity (our inherent interconnectedness) and truth.

> The purpose of violence is to control others, to have them do what they would not otherwise have done, and it does this through physical force, meting out punishment and pain for noncompliance or resistance. As such, targets of violence are denied an independent will and remain targets until they desist in their opposition and comply with the demands of the violent agent [Terchek 2001, 225].

Along these lines, Gandhi envisioned *ahimsa* as both an *avoidance* of causing harm and an *active* form of love that promoted well-being. Gandhi saw love as the "identification with and service of all living beings" (Parekh 1988, 200). For him it was not an argument for the fundamental difference between existing creatures (physical or cultural diversity) but a universal conceptualization of sameness that included all life, "Gandhian love builds on an openness that enables a person to find a unity and mutuality with others.... Gandhian love is expected to be totalizing" (Terchek 2001, 227). Gandhian *ahimsa* is an ethical practice that perceives of a *unity* or an interconnectedness of life. It results in a decrease in interpersonal hostility because it forms a projection outward of positive regard that disarms adversaries. Gandhi was implying "that the power of love brings patience (as a mother has for a recalcitrant child). This patience is required to move the other to see that violence does not necessarily bring about peace," the act of patience is an act of love (Coates 2008, 139–140).

While all violence cannot be eradicated, Gandhian *ahimsa* is committed to loving, nonviolent discipline because it not only transformed the politics of the day; it transformed the people who struggled against violence. For Gandhi "an unshakable faith in the power of truth, love, and suffering, leading to one's own self-transformation, is a prerequisite to sustained non-violent action in the service of the common good" (Bharadwaj 1998, 80). As we will see, pragmatic nonviolence holds no such assertion.

Pragmatic Nonviolence

As considered earlier, there are two general orientations of nonviolence that contain the practice and disciplines of non-harming action: principled nonviolence and pragmatic nonviolence. Pragmatic (or strategic) nonviolence is distinct from what is called principled nonviolence because of its internal or moral dimension. While pragmatic nonviolence aims to socially transform conflict, principled nonviolence (including Gandhian *ahimsa*) results in a transformation of self. Principled nonviolence is associated with pacifism and ethical constraints against the usage of violence, whereas pragmatic nonviolence "refers to a distinctive set of political practices that do not require actors to adopt pacifism" (Howes 2013, 428). Simply put, pacifism and principled nonviolence eschew acts of violence whereas pragmatic nonviolence uses nonviolent acts of protest and resistance to achieve social change.

The major proponent of pragmatic nonviolence is Dr. Gene Sharp (1973). Although Sharp was influenced by the work of Gandhi, and he acknowledges the important nonviolent struggles of Gandhi and of Dr.

Two. Peace Education as Cultural Nonviolence

Martin Luther King, he sees their principled nonviolence as both atypical historically and unnecessary models when seeking to achieve social transformation. Sharp sees nonviolent action as a political tool that requires neither ethical nor spiritual moralities. Indeed, Sharp's approach to nonviolence may be considered superior at recruiting nonviolent activists as a result of the ideological lacunae (Sharp 2005; Weber 2003).

The theory of pragmatic nonviolence (Sharp 1973) focuses on social/political power and using nonviolent action as a tactic to destabilize and co-opt power. Sharp's theory does not seek to recruit or convert political opponents so much as to defeat them. Pragmatic nonviolent activists need not hold personal beliefs that violence is wrong as long as they do not engage in violence to secure power.

> Non-violent struggle is identified by what people do, not what they believe. In many cases, the people using these non-violent methods have believed violence to be perfectly justified in moral or religions terms. However, for the specific conflict that they currently faced they chose, for pragmatic reasons, to use methods that did not include violence [Sharp 2005, 19].

Pragmatic nonviolence, what Sharp terms nonviolent struggle or nonviolent action, uses nonviolence because it works—not because it is morally superior to the use of violence (Weber 2003). Indeed, Sharp conceives of the term nonviolence as problematic because it can be confused with the ethical, moral or religious understandings generally understood to be associated with nonviolence.

> The use of the term "nonviolence" is especially unfortunate, because it confuses these forms of mass action with beliefs in ethical or religious nonviolence ("Principled nonviolence"). Those beliefs, which have their merits, are different phenomena that usually are unrelated to mass struggles conducted by people who do not share such beliefs [Sharp 2005, 20–21].

Pragmatic nonviolence (nonviolent struggle or action) is a method for social transformation based on actions that are either forms of nonviolent protest, persuasion, non-cooperation or nonviolent intervention (Sharp 2005). The theory of nonviolent struggle asserts that true power resides in the hands of ordinary people, not elites and that to take power away from political opponents it is necessary to isolate and remove social groups that uphold political power. This is because by cooperating with a system of government you act to perpetuate it, but by withdrawing your compliance you deteriorate the social "pillars" that sustain the regime. By systematically (and nonviolently) undermining social pillars (security forces, religious organizations, the education system or the media, for example) the consent of the people (the source of political power) is removed and social transformation (social revolution in most instances) results (Sharp 1973).

Cultural Nonviolence

If cultural violence makes direct and structural violence "look, even feel, right—or at least not wrong" then cultural *nonviolence* makes direct and structural violence look, even feel, wrong—or at least not right (Galtung 1990: 291). When Galtung conceived of cultural violence, he also suggested its negation.

> If the opposite of violence is peace, the subject matter of peace research/peace studies, then the opposite of cultural violence would be "cultural peace," meaning aspects of a culture that serve to justify and legitimize direct peace and structural peace. If many and diverse aspects of that kind are found in a culture, we can refer to it as a "peace culture" [Galtung 1990, 291].

Although Galtung negates *cultural violence* with *cultural peace*, recent scholarship and inquiry into the utilization and incarnations of nonviolence (Stephan and Chenoweth 2008; Clements 2008) suggest that there may be something theoretical to gain in leaving the conceptual instability of the word "peace" (defining peace is as problematic for some as defining health or happiness) and using the more commonly defined concept of nonviolence.

Galtung averred that, when aspects that contribute to positive peace exist within a culture, they might be termed "peace culture[s]" (1990, 291). However, earlier, in the same article, Galtung affirms that while there are violent "aspects" within cultures "entire cultures can hardly be classified as violent" (1990, 291). By this rationale "peace cultures" are as unlikely as "violence cultures" and therefore, when we are describing cultural (symbolic) practices that are "aspects" of a culture, we should be aware that, although cultural "aspects" are not held by "entire" populations, they do contribute to the shared symbolic landscape.

When Paolo Freire spoke about the connectivity between reflection and action, he perceived of an equation that recognized that in the social world humans did not exist in silence but instead gave symbolic meaning to authentic interaction (dialogue) through the act of naming the world (word=work=praxis). To Freire, the reflection/action link is critical—should *action* be sacrificed, the result would be verbalism, or idle chatter and, should *reflection* be sacrificed, the result was activism, action without commitment (2003, 87). The act of separating action and reflection negates transformation. Transformation is an internal process that leads to full humanity—humility, trust and hope (Freire 2003). While the word peace can denote a positive reality, the word nonviolence implies an authentic interaction between reflection and action. If we say that cultural violence is an "aspect" of culture that legitimizes direct and structural forms of violence, then we should, equally, be able to say that cultural *nonviolence* are "aspects" of culture that delegitimize direct and structural forms of violence.

Assessing CNV

In Galtung's article, *Cultural Violence* (1990), he observed the connectivity between forms of violence in a violence triangle, "violence can start at any corner in the direct-structural-cultural violence triangle and is easily transmitted to the other corners" (see Figure 1) (302).

By this same reasoning, it might be perceived that cultural *nonviolence* can also emerge from direct-structural-cultural vertices and be transmitted accordingly (see Figure 2).

For instance, structural *nonviolence* could result from punitive legal structures that make acts of physical aggression illegal leading to increases in not only incidences of direct *nonviolence* but symbolic backing for the legal prohibition through religious or scientific support (cultural *nonviolence*).

To determine cultural violence, Galtung posits that "the logic of the scheme is simple: identify the cultural element and show how it can, empirically or potentially, direct of structural violence" (1990, 296). When we utilize this same logic, cultural *nonviolence* should be identifiable by showing how it authentically or theoretically can be used to *delegitimize* direct or structural violence. In order to assess whether

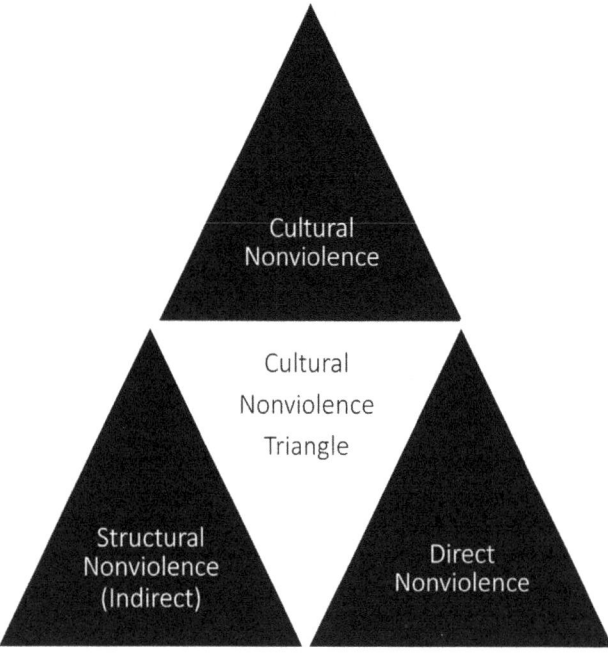

FIGURE 1
Galtung's Violence Triangle (1990)

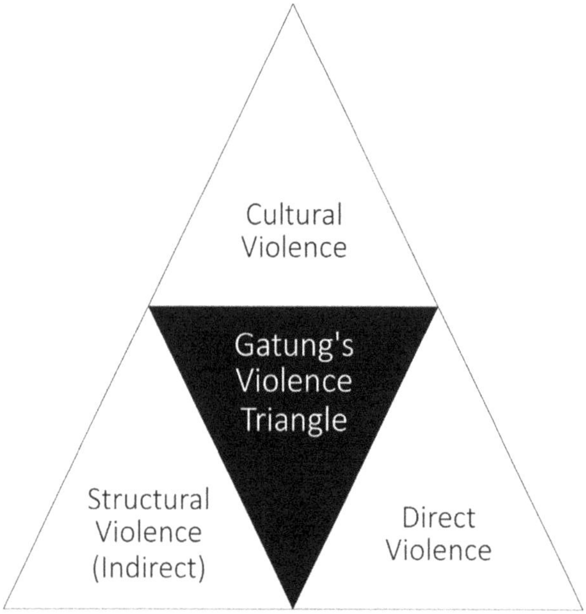

FIGURE 2
The Cultural Nonviolence Triangle (Standish 2014)

Gandhian *ahimsa* and pragmatic nonviolence comprise cultural *nonviolence*, the following questions could be asked:

- Does this cultural "aspect" delegitimize direct violence?
- Does this cultural "aspect" delegitimize structural violence?

After investigating both of these questions it should be relatively easy to discern whether an "aspect" of culture can be considered to be a form of cultural *nonviolence* (see Table 2).

TABLE 2
Cultural Nonviolence

Practice	Delegitimizes Direct Violence	Delegitimizes Structural Violence	Delegitimizes Cultural Nonviolence
Gandhian *ahimsa*	✓	✓	✓
Pragmatic nonviolence	✓	x	x

The practice of Gandhian *ahimsa* can be considered a form of cultural *nonviolence* because, in addition to the ideological prohibition on doing harm to others, the practice directly confronts structural, discriminatory aspects of violence through its unitary vision of life. Pragmatic nonviolence, while it proscribes the use of violence to achieve social transformation, does not delegitimize structural violence. Pragmatic nonviolence is an instrument of political transformation and does not ontologically entertain conditions of inequality. Pragmatic nonviolence is a strategy to defeat one's opponents, not to connect with them. Gandhian *ahimsa*, while it, likewise, eschews the use of force (*himsa*) to achieve social transformation, it also identifies an essential unity of living things that delegitimizes direct and structural violence and therefore can be considered a form of cultural *nonviolence*.

Peace Education as Cultural Nonviolence

Using analogous logic, we should be able to *see* cultural *nonviolence* by asking how it authentically or theoretically can be used to *delegitimize* direct or structural violence. In order to assess whether peace education is a form of cultural *nonviolence* the following two questions are asked:

- Does peace education delegitimize direct violence?
- Does peace education delegitimize structural violence?

The discipline of peace education can be considered a form of cultural nonviolence because it is an aspect of culture (educational culture) that both delegitimizes direct violence and delegitimizes structural violence. If Peace education is a technique used in organized learning to encompass values and practices that aim to decrease or inhibit violence and contribute to peace (Harris and Morrison 2013), then peace education is a form of cultural nonviolence.

> KATERINA: if you ask people to actively engage with their reality you always end up with (unique) impressions of experience and perception: disparate notions of truth, knowledge, perspective, unseen or deliberately hidden information and the impermanence and fallibility of memory, imagination and our emotions. But when you ask "what is in my cultural toolbox" people are not always interested in unpacking that box—a box whose contents are reflected and fortified by our actions, words and thoughts. What do we do when we see something in our cultural toolboxes (containers of who we are, what we believe and what we have been exposed to) that does not resonate with us, or resonate with us "anymore?" What do we take for granted? In my cultural toolbox the "fear" of making a scene engendered all kinds of repression and bottling up of real, genuine emotion. But in my cultural toolbox I also had (sitting directly beside the "repression" center of course) this spicy Mediterranean permission slip to wave my hands and explode once in a while. I had a sense that my emotions were valid and legitimate but at the same time, inappropriate and a sign of weakness. Cultural nonviolence to me relates to more than meta-narratives of living that enshrine values and ideological (or at least functional) capacities but smaller things like humor, solidarity, forgiveness. Traditions have to start somewhere right?
>
> JANINE: Maybe I can share a humorous story that happened during my eighteen months as a foreigner in India. Like any previous classical Yogic researcher I was both the object and subject of the experiment. I was developing a deeper awareness and sensitivity to the world around me. I was lucky in that I spent so much time by myself and for most of that time I did not speak a great deal as my strong kiwi accent was hard for others to understand. And so I listened, experienced and observed more deeply than I had before. It happened when I was reflecting deeply on the practice of ahimsa and its practical utility. I was curious about what the bounds of such a practice could be for myself. I wrote a funny story, in the form of a letter, about a small observation that I had while I was settling into a new environment, community and culture:

Two. Peace Education as Cultural Nonviolence

Dearest Browning children and related and unrelated whanau,

Aunty has been a little busy and sometimes a story can't be forced—it has to emerge in its own time and its own way. Often the things that emerge like that are the very best gift that nature can give us.

Over the last few weeks there have been lots of babies born ... baby cows, baby goats and baby dogs. Aunty tried to befriend a puppy but puppy was very confused by the idea.

However nature always provides and Aunty was given a pet. It was the kind of pet that Aunty never ever imagined herself with. Not really exotic but it kind of had a big nose and I think big eyes and maybe two legs. A very melodic high-pitched song and a devoted nature. At least that was my guess!

My pet arrived unexpectedly the early hours of one morning.

That was a little out of the ordinary however Aunty met her pet at about 4 a.m. in the morning and to begin with she didn't realise that she had a new friend.

Actually it took a couple of mornings.

Now Aunty was finding it hard to wake up in time for morning meditation and her pet started to wake her every morning at the same time. Her friend had a very high voice and endearing habit of blowing air on to her face.

Do you know what kind of pet I was given???

Yep, a pet mosquito.

Yep, I can imagine your surprise but probably not as much as mine.

This mosquito never bit me just woke me at the same time every morning.

There were two in the room one with a deep buzz (not a friend and very happy to bite me) and this other one who would just come and wake me, buzz around my ear, flap her wings fast so there was air on my face and sometimes sit in my head. She would not bite and then would fly away.

This happened every morning for one week and I started to be able to wake naturally for meditation again.

Once I stopped expecting her to bite me, assuming the worst about her. And lets not to mention wanting to kill her.... I realized that mosquitos have different tones to their voice. I always thought they sounded the same. They also somehow feel different.

You know friends like this mosquito need to be treasured because you never know how long they will be with you.

So Aunty learned that friends can come in all sizes and where you least expect them. Aunty used to be scared of mosquitos because her thought was "they will bite me" but sometimes they don't and when you stop being frightened all sorts of unexpected treasures can come.

Today the girls and I went shopping and I happened to say that I needed to get an alarm clock. They burst out laughing and said "But what about your pet mosquito Aunty?" I said: "well you know her life was short and no other mosquito has chosen to befriend me yet!"

Conclusions

All forms of violence, whether direct or structural in nature, have cultural roots. Likewise, many forms of nonviolence can be said to emerge from a shared sense of symbolic significance. This chapter has suggested that in addition to looking at why culture makes certain forms of violence permissible, there is something to be gained by investigating the functional opposite of cultural violence. Put simply (in an inversion of Galtung's notion of cultural violence), how does culture make certain forms of violence impermissible, illegitimate and wrong? And, importantly, how does the way we learn contribute to making violence wrong—or at least not right? The increasingly globalized world and the encounter of other cultures represent an opportunity to increase the human potential for peace by sharing ways of seeing, being and behaving that are based on celebrating and manifesting peace—competencies for the betterment of all life on earth. Surveying cultural *nonviolence* is a way of looking for peace in a sea of conflict. Practicing peace education is a way of building peace.

PART II

YOGIC SCIENCE

THREE

What Is Yoga?

Introduction

Yoga is much more than a fitness class at your local recreation center. Yoga is in fact a nuanced and holistic metaphysical concept and discipline of living. It is essentially the task of becoming a fully integrated human being where one is able to consciously balance one's internal physiological, emotional, relational and spiritual states that may be experienced as an inner physiological awareness and coherence. Its base is a deep and profound capacity to let go, deeply relax and surrender to the subtle forces contained within oneself. It is these subtle energetic forces that Yoga classifies as "love." Yoga is the Sanskrit word meaning "to yoke" or "join" to this inner relational awareness of "love." This notion exists at quite a distance from current popular Yoga practice. As Burley states:

> The term is widely known today, having become entangled with a vast industry. Not only can Yoga classes be found in gyms, sports clubs, colleges, community centers, and village halls throughout the Western world—and elsewhere—but there are also many companies specializing in Yoga equipment, clothing, books, magazines, DVDs, CDs, holidays, and other paraphernalia. Yoga is commercial [and] corporate [2014, 204].

What can this kind of Yoga offer to the field of peace education? Very little it would seem. We are aware that when people are asked to define Yoga, they usually answer that it is a series of exercises or *asana* poses aimed to increase flexibility and suppleness. This is not untrue. Yet, classical Yoga is a non-religious science comprising eight interrelated practices that include attitudes and moral observances, physical *asana* poses and breathing, exteriorization of mind, concentration, meditation or absorption and *samadhi* (translated as bliss or ecstasy in English). Each of these practices builds upon the others, with the attitudes and moral observances acting as the stable platform and base. Throughout this chapter, we will present an integrated, practical understanding and definition according to these eight aspects of classical Yoga and, in doing so; we will draw on research from the fields of neuro-psycho-biology, physiology, psychology, and philosophy.

Lost in Translation

Yoga is a manageable and rigorous discipline. Understanding Yoga is a journey that means acquiring knowledge that is part cognitive (you don't know until you *learn* it) and part experiential (you don't know until you have *done* it). A further challenge relates to the use of abstract language where the language of Yoga (Sanskrit) does not easily translate into other languages. Translations from Sanskrit into English have presented some difficulties given English's lack of deep varied terms for matters of inner consciousness and spirituality. The *Bhagavad-gita* describes Yoga as:

> Let this be known by the name of Yoga, this viYoga (disconnection) from samYoga (firm vision) with duhkhu (sorrow or pain)—where in the citta (mental being) restrained by Yoga-seva (Yogic practices) comes to rest, wherein one beholds the Cosmic Self through his individual self and rejoices in the Cosmic Self, wherein one experiences that supreme bliss that can be grasped by the buddhi (pure intellect), but is beyond the reach of the senses wherein established one does not deviate from the truth. On gaining which one cannot conceive of any greater gain than that and where in anchored one is not shaken even by the heaviest duhkha (sorrow or pain) [20–23, in Radhakrishnan 1974].

However valuable the concepts and teachings within the *Bhagavad-gita* are, words such as *buddhi* are not easily understood (much less understood deeply) unless the phenomena they name have been experienced personally. This is one of the key difficulties of this Yogic Science. If these inner conditions have not been personally experienced and developed, then an individual remains ignorant of the other deeper levels of awareness and neural integration.

One of the world's best known peace educators, Mahatma Gandhi, described his own integration of spiritual and practical awareness thusly: "I believe in non-duality, I believe in the essential unity of man and, for that matter, of all that lives.... The rock-bottom foundation of the technique for achieving the power of nonviolence is belief in the essential oneness of all life" (Gandhi 1924, 390). Our experience of an integrated approach towards the awareness of unity and essential oneness of life is not solely extraordinary. It has flowed from practices that have developed an inner subtle condition of awareness, unity, balance, connection and love. We agree with Gandhi that this integrated consciousness may give the capacity for increased tolerance, and creative nonviolence. However, it may not develop a complete or saintly relational ethics, as Gandhi himself demonstrated in his own controversial attempts to remain spiritually pure while sleeping alongside young women (Gier and Ranganathan 2007). While the integrated consciousness may be described as a space where ordinary ego reactions are more easily observed, managed and transformed, it does not guarantee that the individual will practice discipline in their outer behaviors. Perhaps such a total discipline is not possible or even desirable for human beings. Janine has this to add:

> JANINE: Forty-two years after my first introduction to yogic practices; I can experience words such as Cosmic Self, buddhi, supreme bliss as both meaningful and a bit nonsensical. The words don't really describe the condition properly and I still can't find the words in English that do. Perhaps it is really trying to describe what is essentially indescribable and natural. It feels beyond experience and for me is more of an inner condition or balance. That's why it seems silly to try and define it. However, when I used to try to understand this integration logically and cognitively through my mind, there were thoughts about definition, doubt, exceptional religious standards of cosmic self, expectations of otherworldly experiences and inner confusion. This approach seldom led me to any neural integration or peaceful centered experience. Later as my yogic practice deepened it transformed into an inner feeling from a contemplative inner heart space. It seems then that my whole physiological and emotional system relaxed into a different subtle consciousness. There was some kind of an inner and outer congruence, integration within me. From this space there was an ordinary awareness of connection with all forms of life. At times this was observable as an expanded experience of love, compassion and knowledge. At that stage it depended upon my inner steadiness and willingness to be still. You know, relaxed and silent on the inside, not reacting, just resting within presence. Later those states and conditions were no longer observable. Perhaps they had become natural within me. I can now behave without discipline on the outside but I am less willing to. I don't pretend that it

is different to what it is. If it is greedy then it is greedy. This is all. An opportunity to be grateful and readjust, retune and realign.

KATERINA: I could not agree more—these talents of truthful observation lead to the clarity. And they are talents anyone can develop. You speak about how your "whole physiological and emotional system relaxed into a different subtle consciousness" and that is literally my sense of how yogic practices lead you to a feeling of both concrete stillness and energetic lightness. For me there is a deeply rooted sense that seems to effortlessly exist simultaneously with a feeling of fearless detachment. The recognition of the illusions leads to a lovely feeling of grateful confidence. You say "you don't pretend it is different than it is" and that comfort with reality is really a lifted burden. Seeing things as they are, myself as I am, leads to that pleasant "that is all" feeling and I find that simplicity exquisite.

Generally, classical Yoga does not encourage blind belief; rather it offers a range of practices that others have found useful in preparing their physiological systems for the experience of awareness and first-hand knowledge of union and connectivity. For most human beings, our lives are not a belief, nor are they a science; rather our lives are a creative art; the creative art of choosing our inner and outer response to the external challenges facing us. Or perhaps we react automatically without inner awareness. Whenever an individual has developed a deep integration we find examples in their ordinary lives of transformation, creative projects and spontaneous happenings, even in situations where there is danger, repression, loss and suffering.

According to Yogic Science, each human being has the capacity to develop a consciousness that generates a deep condition of connection with life, vitality and unity. From this base a relational ethics and capacity to live respectfully with others develops. Brantmeier (2007) describes this natural way of being in the following words:

> Thus, non-violent action in the world begins with loving oneself, extending that love to others, and acting without a seam between non-violent thought and non-violent action. The spontaneous flow of love becomes inherent in every action. With a "recognition of the fundamental unity of all life" we move forward with loving kindness [137].

As we reflect on this passage it seems that the key word is "spontaneously." Brantmeier (2007) describes a natural outpouring of love that expresses itself in the lives of the human beings as a relational, unified ethics. Yoga and all other contemplative traditions have valued this transformative and peaceful capacity of each human being.

Throughout this chapter we will attempt to simplify your understanding of Yoga while referencing experimental outcome studies. We will also identify the benefits that yogic practices are having in the classroom and in the wider community. As we write these words we are reminded of a recent high school student social media post. It goes like this: a young person is sitting looking forlorn with the written caption, "I am feeling anxious. I am feeling depressed." In the next picture her friends are seated in a cheerful group chanting "Yoga, Yoga, Yoga." Any of us who have relaxed deeply in a Yoga *asana* or meditation class will know that sense of light-weight wellbeing. It really is very nice and this short reprieve from day-to-day tension has led to a current wave of popularity for *Hatha Yoga* (the practice of *asana* poses and *pranayama*) and meditation. However, the discipline of Yoga is not a cure-all, nor a magical path towards utopian peace. Rather it is a disciplined series of practices that eventually lead to a natural "moment by moment" responsiveness to life and the capability to both choose and embody balance. It is not a "one size fits all" approach to life, nor does it lie within the realm of mass social movements or religion. Janine speaks about her experience gaining yogic knowledge:

> As the fortunate recipient of a Commonwealth scholarship that involved living and studying at a traditional Sanskrit University, I was able to gain access to the biographies of many Yoga practitioners. What surprised my Western mind was that, in general, the classical teachers saw no difference between inner and outer peace. It was natural that meditational and effective yogic practices led to service and works that benefited the wider community. Many had stories whereby they critiqued unjust social traditions and worked to break down racial, religious and gender inequalities. Traditionally teachers and students lived together in families and developed a relational ethics. The teacher found the correct way to teach according to the nature and mind of the student.

Katerina, walking a very different path, remarks,

> My path was almost an inverse of your experience. In my case, the teachers that I studied with were lacking the holisticism you describe, and who I was or how I learned was immaterial. When I began Yoga in the West there was no community of practitioners for me and the only opportunity that I had to briefly glimpse that wellbeing or find a space or as you say "reprieve" from the day-to-day came in class. My first exposures to Yoga discipline were fragmented (a flow class here, an Iyengar class there and a bit of Kundalini thrown in to make things diverse) but still, the practice itself began to make me feel integrated. When you speak about your teachers and how they did not feel a separateness between, as you say, "inner

and outer peace" this is completely opposite to my experience where the only opportunity to practice Yoga for me was on the mat. Those of us who first found Yoga on our mats need to understand how much more yogic practices have to transform our inner and outer worlds.

Peaceful People Create Peaceful Communities

Well-regarded Indian teacher-scientist-practitioners, such as Patanjali, Vivekananda, Ramakrishna, OSHO, and Abhadananda, have viewed Yoga as the ultimate science concerned with the development of human beings with a natural peaceful and balanced consciousness; the place of humanity within an interconnected ecosystem; and the interplay of subtle forces and matter. They have each expressed deep concern about the state of human life and in particular the levels of violence and harm. They each have focused upon questions of individual evolution and peaceful community. They concluded that a yogic lifestyle created individuals with inner psychological steadiness and calm, which in turn created responsible, peaceful communities. They maintained a non-religious perspective. Throughout this book we will review the literature to see how these practical experiences of yogic community have utility within the field of peace education.

Classical Definitions of Yoga

Yoga is the Sanskrit language term, which reflects the yoking and joining of consciousness, seen in the two words from which "Yoga" is derived. The first root word, *yujir*, means unity, union, connection, intimacy and harmony. The second Sanskrit root word is *yuj*, which means to control and to contemplate. Maharishi Patanjali was the first researcher to codify and compile all the practices of Yoga[1] and his work is considered an authoritative and integrated account of Yoga philosophy, psychology and physiological practices (Prasada 1912; Ananthuraman 1996; Feuerstein 2001). He described Yoga as: "Yogas citta vritti nirodha." This can be transcribed from the Sanskrit into English as: "Yoga as the state of cessation *(norodha)* of all fluctuations (*vrittis*) in the mental being or the inner instrument of cognition and consciousness (*citta*)" (Prabhavananda 2012, Yoga Sutra, 1, 2). Another ancient

Indian text, the Katha Upaniṣhad, defined Yoga as "Tam Yogam-iti manyante sthiram-indriya-dharanam," which is transcribed from the Sanskrit into English as: "The highest state is, they say, when the five senses of knowledge, together with the manas (the lower mental faculty) cease from their normal activities and the buddhis (pure intellect) itself does not stir. This, they consider to be the state of Yoga, this firm holding back of the senses, when one is completely undistracted. Yoga, verily, is beginning and end (or birth and death)" (Katha Upaniṣhad, II, 3.II).

How can we understand these words given our current state of knowledge? It is useful to recall that both the goal and meaning of Yoga are union, which is ultimately achieved through processes of meditation and *samadhi*. From this perspective we can choose to understand the Katha Upaniṣhad words according to the electrical activity and functional activities within the brain. Recent studies have examined the effects of Satyananda Yoga meditation practice on electroencephalogram (EEG) measures (Thomas, Jamieson and Cohen, 2014) by using eLORETA (exact standardized low resolution electromagnetic tomography) to compare differences in cortical source activity, underlying scalp EEG intermediate (mean experience: 4 years) and advanced (mean experience: 30 years).

Australian meditators from the Satyananda Yoga tradition were studied during a body-steadiness meditation, mantra meditation, and during non-meditation. Intermediate Yoga meditators showed greater source activity at low frequencies (particularly theta and alpha1). Advanced Yoga meditators showed greater activity at high frequencies (beta and especially gamma) in all conditions but these were greatly expanded during meditation practice. Here we can see similarities to the increased gamma frequencies that have been observed in advanced Buddhist meditators and are associated with an increased compassionate response to suffering (Brefczynski, Lutz, Schaefer, Levinsky and Davidson 2007; Condon, Desbordes, Miller and Deston 2013). It is possible that we would see similar changes in those following Christian and Muslim contemplative practices. A recent meta-analysis by Boccio, Piccardi and Guariglia (2015) found that meditation in general led to increased functional activation in brain areas, including the bilateral middle frontal gyrus; precentral gyrus; anterior cingulate cortex; insula; and the claustrum. In the left hemisphere they found increased activation of the inferior frontal gyrus; precuneus; caudate nucleus; and the thalamus; and in the right hemisphere increased activation in the: medial frontal gyrus; parahippocampal gyrus; middle occipital gyrus; inferior parietal lobule; and the lentiform nucleus.

According to the *Bhagavad-gita,* Yoga is defined as "Samatvam Yogamuchyate" (Radhakrishnan, 1974, II, 48) which translates into English as "being stable." While there is a range of yogic practices according to the eight stages of development, the constant state of *samadhi* is the ultimate outcome of union. It does not surprise us that researchers are discovering that different meditation techniques require different cognitive processes and show different neural effects (Hölzel, Ott, Hempel, Hackl, Wolf, Stark and Vaitl 2007; Boccio, Piccardi and Guariglia 2015). In general however, meditation practice is viewed as a process that involves the capacity to experience detachment from one's thoughts; the capacity to regulate attention; and the ability to induce relaxation states. Perhaps these are the capacities that are inherent when one is able to practice Yoga, as described by the *Bhagavad-gita,* as "*viYoga* (disconnection) from *samYoga* (firm vision) with *duhkha* (sorrow or pain)." The references to Cosmic self and supreme bliss are perhaps a little more difficult to connect with current neurological findings. However, Lehmann, Faber, Tei, Pascual-Marqui, Milz and Kochi (2012) remind us that all meditation traditions have been interested in:

> The handling of the contents of consciousness (avoiding intruding unintended thoughts as described as in terms such as e.g. letting go, benevolent disregard, detachment), and the quality of the conscious self-awareness (attaining a pleasant, peaceful state of mind as described in terms such as all-oneness, bliss, oceanic feeling, transcending, expanded consciousness) [2012, 1575].

Their study examined the EEG topographies of experienced meditators in five traditions (Tibetan Buddhists (n=13), *QiGong* (n=15), Sahaja Yoga (n=14), Ananda Yoga (n=14), and Zen (n=15)). They found that there was no difference between the traditions, as the optimal meditation state for all was characterized by reduced intra-cortical functional connectivity compared to no-task resting (Lehman et al. 2012). Their findings suggest that the reduced connectivity between brain regions may help us to understand the deep yogic experiences described by the *Bhagavad-gita,* "wherein one beholds the Cosmic Self through his individual self and rejoices in the Cosmic Self, wherein one experiences that supreme bliss that can be grasped by the *buddhi* (pure intellect)" (Bhagavad-gita, VI, in Radhakrishnan, 1974, 20–23).

What seems clear from the ancient definitions of Yoga and current neurological research is that the optimal experience of yogic consciousness leads to changes in the mind of the human being. The yogic classical text, Patanjali's *Yoga Sutras*, describes the eight limbs leading to such change as ethics (*yama*); restraints (*niyama*); poses (*asana*); energy control (*pranayama*); interiorization of the mind (*pratyahara*); concentration (*dharana*); meditation or absorption (*dhyana*); and oneness/blissful condition (*samadhi*). In this coding system, various yogic scientists have systematically recorded each aspect of practice and its effects. Patanjali outlines their method of inquiry in sutra 1: "Direct observation, rational inference and verbal cognition (or recorded testimony) constitutes the sources of right knowledge" (*Pratyaksanumanagamah pramanani*) (Ananthuraman 1996, 27). The outcomes of practice were systematized and replicated from teacher to student prior to Patanjali's codification system.

Four Yogic Pathways

Prominent teacher and social activist Swami Vivekânanda identified different pathways of Yoga suitable to differing human natures: union through mysticism suits the *Raja Yogi*; union through love and devotion is called *bhakti Yogi*; union through philosophy suits the *jnana Yogi*; and union through selfless service suits the *karma Yogi* (Vivekânanda 1923; Abhedananda 1967). Some human beings take a more integrated pathway, which involves all four aspects. Regardless of the path chosen, it is said that all Yoga pathways lead to Raja Yoga, while the practice of Raja Yoga solely creates the normalization of *asana* posture, breathing, purification, service and devotion necessary for reaching the goal (Prasada 1912; Feuerstein 2001; Ananthuraman 1996). Yoga throughout this book is understood as a complete lifestyle practice that includes a holistic and personalized application of the eight aspects of Yogic Science.

Yoga as an integration of practices can lead to a change of relational, ethical and consciousness paradigms in its practitioners (Adhia et al. 2010; Feuerstein 2001; Rajagopalachari 2013; Travis and Pearson 2000). However, Patanjali's *Yoga sutra* (3:6) *asana, Tasya bhumisu viniyapath*, indicates that the application of Yoga techniques should be according to the constitution of the individual. Every single human being is unique and therefore the application of Yoga should be individualized. This is a very useful point and one that we will remain aware of as we enter the chapters describing the specific techniques that have applicability in peace education and in the classroom. It can be difficult to identify which technique or pathway is suitable to each person. It requires careful observation of the student's mind-set in a range of settings. Traditionally the Yoga teacher observed and lived alongside the student for periods of time (Abhyankar 2015). This is clearly not possible for modern yogic peace educators. However, we can encourage the depth of inner observation, reflection and awareness such that the student can make informed and disciplined choices about the most suitable pathway for their constitution.

Raja Yoga Pathway

The Sanskrit word *raja* translates as "king." Raja Yoga is therefore the "King of Yoga" and is a "method of mental regulation." It is comprised of *dharana*/concentration, *dhyana*/meditation and *samadhi*/bliss. Modern forms of Raja Yoga exist which are said to offer these teachings in a manner more suitable to the modern mind, which is less religious and more secular. Patanjali's traditional *yama*/restraints include: (i) non-injury, (ii) truthfulness, (iii) non-stealing, and (iv) being greedless; and the *niyama*/observances or values: (i) purity, (ii) contentment, (iii) asceticism, (iv) self-study, and (v) surrender to *Ishwara*/supreme being or cosmic consciousness, form the base of classical Raja Yoga (see Table 3).

According to Patanjali, these *yama* and *niyama*, alongside physiological and meditational effects and practice, form an interconnected base for a consciousness of unity. The practice of individual restraint include *ahimsa* (non-injury), *satyam* (truthfulness), *asteyam* (non-stealing), *brahmacharya* (chastity/moderation) and *aparigraha* (greedlessness) (Prabhavananda 2012).

Some theorists suggest that adhering to *yama* and *niyama* increases a sense of connectedness between people—the reduction of self-interest

TABLE 3
Yama and Niyama

Restraints (Yama)	Observances (Niyama)
Non-injury *(ahimsa)*	Purity or cleanliness *(shaucha)*
Truthfulness *(satya)*	Contentment *(santosha)*
Non-stealing *(asteya)*	Asceticism or austerity *(tapas)*
Chastity *(brahmacharya)*	Self-study *(swadhyaya)*
Greedlessness *(aparigraha)*	Devotion to Spirit *(ishwara-pranidhana)*

heightening workers' morality (Corner 2009). According to Yoga scientist Satyananda (1976), "The yamas may extend our knowledge of connectedness, a central principle in workplace spirituality, because these are practices that deepen awareness of connection with others and provide insight into the broad social environment" (378).

In this way, the *yama* and *niyama* become values, attitudinal and behavioral practices that may attune our awareness towards a relational, hospitable experience of each other. Thus they may have utility beyond bloodlines and friendship and towards a universal way of relating regardless of our personalities and identities. In the following section we examine the individual *yama* and *niyama* in more detail.

YAMA

The *yamas* are restraints on personal conduct and include the yogic ethics of *ahimsa, satya, asteya, brahmacharya and aparigraha.*

Ahimsa

Ahimsa is the practice of non-harming and has been generally defined as, "not injuring others by thought, word or deed" (Vivekânanda 1899, 295). It is the first listed individual restraint or capacity to be developed. In its strictest manifestation, it is the dictate to not kill or be violent towards others, including all forms of animal, plant and mineral life. An individual who is practicing *ahimsa*, in the context of modern *Yoga*, is likely to employ an expanded perspective (Holcombe

2015). For example, *ahimsa* may include being prudent in the use of nature's resources, which shows integration with the observance of *aparigraha* (greedlessness). However, while it is possible for most human beings to aspire to a life-caring or life-nourishing practice, it is impossible to not harm another living being. Holcombe (2015) helps us understand in the following words, how we may develop a pragmatic moral sensitivity and flexibility in our best effort to not hurt the environment, other living beings and each other:

> II.31 jati desa kala samaya anavicchinna sarvabhaumah mahavratam. In this sutra, Patanjali acknowledges that only those very rare beings in all the worlds (sarvabhaumah) who have taken a "great vow" (mahavratam) are able to practice all five yamas without interruption (vicchinna), while—and this is key—the rest of us must adapt these guidelines to our current occupation (jati), the place we live (desa), time of day, month, or year (kala), or circumstance (samaya) [31].

This sutra recognizes that not many of us are capable of practicing: *ahimsa*/non-injury, *satya*/truthfulness, *asteya*/non-stealing, *brahmacharya*/continence, and *aparigraha*/greedlessness, in a continuous way. Pure *ahimsa* is almost impossible for an individual to practice, given our current system of global production based on systems of inequality, environmental impoverishment and effect on other life forms. Even the act of inhalation destroys microbes. However, if we re-orientate *ahimsa* towards the possibility of achieving a "life-caring" stance, we may be more successful. This stance allows us to be mindful in our use of resources; mindful in the way we exercise our power as global consumers; mindful of what we support and create in our local communities; and, for those of us in democracies, mindful of political power. *Ahimsa* as life caring may create an internal paradigm shift based on possibility rather than intrinsic failure. It recognizes the role that we can have as loving stewards in co-relation with all living beings.

Satya

Satya is the Sanskrit word for truthfulness. It conveys the idea of being truthful and consistent with reality in words, thoughts and actions. It describes a knowing of what is correct once the rationalizations of our minds are stripped away (Corner 2009). At a deeper level truth is the realization of "unity within diversity" and the interconnectedness of all life and the rejection of false perception and communication.

Panduranga (2009) remarks upon the deep attitudes forming the base of a yogic lifestyle:

> The ancient Indians sought fellowship with every living being and the same is expressed in the following hymn of the Yajurveda:
> May all beings look on me with the eye of a friend,
> May I look on all beings with the eye of a friend,
> May we look on one another with the eye of a friend [115].

This attitude of fellowship was viewed as one of the fruits of sincere and regular practice of yogic principles. We suggest that this realization and practice of truth may have modern utility, leading to potential expressions of harmony in relationship. In truth, we build relationships and in lies, we destroy them. The yogic practice of *satya* perceives that only through truth can we speak and be heard with respect, attention and love. This is more than avoiding falsehoods but speaking gently, mindfully and with honesty.

Asteya

Asteya is the Sanskrit word for non-stealing and avoidance of misappropriations in thought and action (Abhyankar 2015). It relates to the yogic ethic of refusing to take what does not belong to you, refusing to take when others go without and refusing to crave the possessions or qualities of others. This is not simply a value that relates to material possessions but also to thoughts, ideas or the outcomes of our ideas. To crave what another possesses is to compare what one has with what belongs to another. A simple act of recognizing how possessions are dissimilar leads to an act of separation (they *have* that and I do not, or vice versa), which is fundamentally at odds with the yogic ethic of interconnectivity. To discern difference in what "you" and "I" possess leads to a false perception that we are different. We are not what we *have*, we are one, and so what belongs to oneself or to another is only a false marker of separateness. The yogic practice of *asteya* reminds us that "I" am not *more than* or *less than* because "I" *have* things (possessions, ideas) and neither are "you."

Brahmacharya

Brahmacharya is the Sanskrit word for moderation or non-wastage of energy. As Corner (2009) describes:

> This yama is often narrowly thought of as sexual continence but it is really broader and applies to all situations of emotional involvement, not just

sexual involvement. A person practicing bramacharya would show discretion and discrimination in all activities leading to emotional involvement with others to avoid the stress that can result from the multiplicity of emotional connections [382].

In many ways this describes an avoidance of the romantic intoxication of intimate relations and an inner discrimination of respectful relationship with the other. The call to practice moderation and self-control encourages ourselves to be humble and conscious of our desires. As this *yama* refers to walking with a "higher self," it reminds us that strict restraint from something can rob us of energy as we focus on maintaining the prohibition of something. The yogic discipline of *bramacharya* reminds us that staying in the middle path—living neither in excess nor in denial—is the option that leads to a greater chance at balance. Being moderate in body, mind and speech emerges from self-awareness of desire and respect for self and others.

Aparigraha

Aparigraha is the Sanskrit word for greedlessness and non-acquisitiveness (Abhyankar, 2015). It recognizes that the *shat ripus*/six foes preventing stable inner health and peace are: (i) *kama*/lust, (ii) *krodha*/anger, (iii) *lobha*/greed, (iv) *manda*/pride or aggression, (v) *moha*/desire, and (vi) *matsar*/jealousy. These were the primary instincts that increased the vulnerability of the individual towards inner preoccupation and poor mental health. The practice of non-acquisitiveness is an aspect of nonviolence because an individual who has their needs met does not burden the planet with over consumption (nor develop stress related illness). According to Panduranga (2009) the practice of *aparigraha* was a key in maintaining an ecological harmony.

> The Vedic seers perceived the value of maintaining a harmonious relationship between the needs of human beings and the spectacular diversity of the universe. To them, nature was not only a mother to sustain their life; it was the abode of divinity. They did not believe that humans' role on Earth was to exploit nature for their own selfish purposes. Nor did they believe in the view that the true end of humans was essentially to dominate and control nature by all possible means. On the contrary, sanctity of life to them included not only the individual efforts to seek salvation but also to achieve it by developing a sacred attitude towards nature and its manifestations. This is evidenced in the sacred concept of deva-yajna in which human beings are asked to worship the Gods who are personifications of various natural phenomena. They had great love and regard for the five

primary elements namely, (1) the earth, (2) the water, (3) the fire, (4) the air and (5) the space, collectively called pancha-mahabhutas. The ancient Indian view of the five elements acknowledges that they are essential for peace, happiness and tranquility in the universe and for the flowering and development of humanity [111].

In choosing to live simply we free ourselves of the burden of possessions and more, allow ourselves to understand that, because our needs are being met, we do not need to waste energy yearning for goods or gratification (we think) we do not have (or do not have yet). In still another sense, the yogic ethic of *aparigraha* allows us to perceive the true abundance in our lives—not the feeling of scarcity that leads to fear and grasping—and this sense of satiety of life leads to feeling safe and gratified. When you feel full you have no need to hoard, accumulate or feel insecure.

NIYAMA

Niyamas are observances or rules of behavior that apply to individual conduct including *saucha, santosha, tapas, swadhyaya* and *ishwara pranidana*.

Saucha

Saucha is the Sanskrit word for cleanliness or purity. At a practical level this refers to the physical body. At another level it refers to the quality of ideas and consciousness in which we associate. Yogic physical practices lead to a clarity of mind and good physiological function, including regulated digestion and bowel function; equal breathing through both nostrils; nervous system resilience; and spinal and musculature strength and flexibility.

Saucha can be separated into internal and external practices where external purity is associated with hygiene and cleanliness whereas internal purity is related to the foods we eat and life-giving quality of balanced, healthful and nutrient rich food. The maxim "you are what you eat" firmly applies in the yogic ethic of *saucha* where the body is conceived of as a vessel for the spirit that must be cared for. The observance of *saucha* also refers to clean thinking where internal cleanliness is associated with cleansing the mind of thoughts that are disturbing or destructive. By observing *saucha* the body becomes healthy, the mind becomes clear and this clarity of mind gives an internal space free of preoccupied, automatic thinking. When we are free from automatic thinking we can perceive of others with love and compassion.

Santosha

Santosha is the Sanskrit word for contentment. This is the deep pleasurable contentment that is mixed with knowledge, gratitude and joy. It is a more accurate way of describing the inner condition, which is a deep steady state. It is not akin to the emotional experience of joy, ecstasy or happiness but rather refers to a feeling of tranquility or gratitude. Feeling content means the mind does not seek out distractions that fuel our desires and, in turn, this contentedness—in seeking nothing, needing nothing—means that our lack of desire for other things inhibits a tendency to compare, contrast and find fault with what is different. This happy-stance permits us to be appreciative of things in a way that reminds us of our non-separateness and allows us to cherish things we commonly take for granted: our friends, our families, our circumstances and ourselves.

Tapas

Tapas is the Sanskrit word for seriousness. This in the context of Yoga means the diligent practice of yogic lifestyle and meditation. Traditionally it was the practice of going and living in an ashram or similar environment for some time and practicing all aspects of Yoga conscientiously. The yogic ethic of *tapas* also refers to the opportunity to practice yogic discipline by "burning" up or cleansing feelings, thoughts or desires that become challenges or obstacles to perceiving the unity of life. By incorporating the *niyama* of *tapas*, a *yogin* builds up character by practicing the yogic lifestyle—this leads to resilience as we continually face challenges that we overcome through the exercise of letting go.

Swadhyaya

Swadhyaya is the Sanskrit word for self-study. It has been understood to include the outer aspect of studying sacred spiritual texts however, it is the inner practice of being able to observe one's inner actions of ego, including: emotional reaction, thoughts, motivations, prejudice and fears. From this observational awareness and self-study the practitioner experiences transformational inner change. It begins with awareness, an inward gaze which leads to knowledge that cultivates compassion, tolerance and objectivity. This then becomes a natural part of the outer personality. The yogic ethic of *swadhyaya* permits the investigation of the divine in the self and the opportunity to recognize the deep interconnectivity present in the universe.

Ishwara pranidhana

Ishwara pranidhana is the Sanskrit phrase meaning devotion, being one with the divine or surrendering towards God's will (Abhyankar 2015). In *ishwara pranidhana* the practitioner's experience of the divine is not defined (no single entity or understanding is preferred) and emerges naturally out of the practice of self-study. It is the progression from the study of the lesser domain (self) to the study of the greater domain (God/god consciousness/universal spirit). The concept of *ishwara* refers to the indeterminate reality behind the objects not accessible to the sense objects or, put another way, *ishwara* can be considered the divine essence in all things not readily observable. The final *niyama* (observance) practices the act of unitary perception—the divine is everywhere, it surrounds us and infuses all matter (Poetic naturalists would describe our cellular connectivity as the nature of reality). The *yogini* who practices *ishwara pranidhana* sees spirit in everything and this observation is an act of devotion as we surrender our hearts, minds and spirit to the divine (the divine is unseeable).

HATHA YOGA PATHWAY

Modern variants of Hatha Yoga are common and can be seen in Sivananda Yoga classes, hot Yoga, Iyengar and Ashtanga Yoga classes. While the teachers in these classes are often trained in all eight branches of classical Yoga, this is not guaranteed. They teach the classical yogic *asana*/posture and third limb of Yogic Science, and variations according to set class routines or according to the body needs of the participants. The classes are weighted towards the physical *asana*/postures, and some *pranayama*/energy control or introductory breathing exercise may be included. *Asana* are concerned with regulating the nervous system in the body such that tension is released and the circulatory, respiratory, skeletal, digestive, elimination, systems function correctly.

Patanjali's *Yoga Sutras* identify the various health effects in the following sutras: (i) mental (2, 2; 1, 32–39), (ii) cause of illness (2, 4; 2, 12), (iii) spiritual health (2, 25–26; 2, 28), (iv) physical health (2, 29; 2: 35–45), and (v) conduct and ethics (2, 30–32) (Prasada 1912). Yogendra Svatmarama, in the 14th century book, *Hatha Yoga Pradipika*, describes specific physical health benefits of *Hatha Yoga*, for example in *Sloka* 2,25: "There is no doubt that coughs, asthma, diseases of the spleen, leprosy and twenty kinds of diseases caused by excess mucus are destroyed through the effects of dhauti karma." Modern research during the last fifty years on the various techniques or methods in Yoga (including breathing, meditation, physical postures, centering, and visualization) has verified many of these ancient findings. Indeed, the list of disorders has expanded to include the amelioration of stress-related mental and physical disorders such as asthma, high blood pressure, cardiac illness, elevated cholesterol, irritable bowel syndrome, cancer, insomnia, multiple sclerosis, and fibromyalgia (Benson 1996; Becker 2000). A review of the literature by Field (2011) noted the positive effects of Yoga poses on psychological conditions including anxiety and depression, on pain syndromes, cardiovascular, autoimmune and immune conditions, and on pregnancy. Further, the physiological effects of Yoga included decreased heart rate and blood pressure. Physical effects included weight loss and increased muscle strength (Sukshole and Phataket 2012).

The classical *asana* poses were developed by adept meditation practitioners to keep the physical body functioning during prolonged periods of inner practice. Most modern Hatha Yoga classes would include the common relaxation and warm up *asana*. *Yoganidra* is a relaxation pose, which is practiced lying prone, and following *sankalpa*, progressive muscle relaxation and visualization. *Shavasana* refers to a relaxation pose that relieves headaches, dizziness, mental weaknesses, insomnia, high blood pressure and sciatica back pain. It improves digestion, balances hormones and relaxes the whole psycho-physiological system. It should ideally be practiced before sleep or before, during and after *asana* such as *Surya Namaskar* (Salute to the Sun).

The *asana* poses taught in any class routine are varied according to the teacher tradition and the needs of the students. Classes may include the following classic *asana*: *shirshasana* (headstand), *sarvangasana* (shoulder stand), *halasana* (plough), *setubandhasana* (bridge), *matsyasana* (fish), *gomukhasana* (cow face), *paschimothanasana* (forward bend), *poorvotanasana* (inclined plane), *bhujangasana* (cobra), *shalabhasana* (locust), *dhanurasana* (bow), *ardha matsyendrasana* (half spinal twist), *kakasana* (crow), *trikonasana* (triangle), *vrikshasana* (tree) and *tadasana* (mountain).

Certain *kriya* or cleansing practices may also be taught. The *Hatha Yoga Pradipika* states that the practice of *nauli* stimulates the digestive fire, thereby removing toxins, indigestion, and constipation. It is considered a *Shat Karma*, which is an internal cleansing process to aid the body that has excess phlegm, mucus, or fat. The *Gheranda Samhita*, which pre-dates the *Hatha Yoga Pradipika*, describes *nauli*, "With great force move the stomach and intestines from one side to the other." It also claims that it destroys all diseases and increases the bodily fire, while toning the abdominal muscles and massaging the internal organs. Mastery of three locks or holds in the body (*Mula, Uddiyana* and *Jalandhara Bandha* locks) is essential in the practice of *nauli*. *Mula bandha* seals vital energy at the level of the perineum (floor of the pelvis), while *Jalandhara bandha* closes the current at the glottis (pit of the throat) so that any of the toxin cleansing heat or energy generated in the torso does not move into the higher centers. The practice of *Uddiyaana* strengthens the abdominal muscles and diaphragm by massaging the abdominal viscera, the solar plexus, heart and lungs. It increases the gastric fire; improves digestion, assimilation and elimination; and purifies the digestive tract of toxins. It stimulates blood circulation in the abdomen and blood flow to the brain. It also stimulates and lifts the energy of the lower belly (*apana vayu*), to unite it with the energies localized in the navel (*samana vayu*) and heart (*prana vayu*).

Bhakti Yoga Pathway

Bhakti Yoga is the process of balance and union through love and devotion towards God. *Bhakti* is the Sanskrit language term describing the attitude of devotion towards a personal God and is experienced as one soul and one super soul. Most Yoga practitioners do not attempt to define God and this pathway does not suit everyone, particularly if one subscribes to an atheist lens.

Bhakti is an ancient practice first referred to in the *Shvetashvatara*

Upanisad and later in the *Bhagavad-gita*. The *Bhagavata Purana* (N.A. [2012] 7.5, 23–24) identifies nine aspects of *bhakti* practice: (i) s*ravana* (listening to stories of Krishna and his companions), (ii) *kirtana* (praise often through group singing), (iii) *visnoh smarana* (remembering or fixing the mind upon the preferred deity), (iv) *pada-sevana* (rendering service), (v) *arcana* (worshipping an image that enables one to remember the preferred deity), (vi) *vandana* (paying homage), (vii) *dasya* (servitude), (viii) *sakhya* (friendship), and (ix) *atma-nivedana* (complete surrender of self).

Practitioners may use the technique of *japa*, which is the repetition of a chosen deity's name and constantly remembering He/She and Her/His form. For non-theists (those who do not perceive of a personal god) or non-deists (those who do not perceive of a divine creator) this maxim may sit uncomfortably. Brantmeier's writing (2007) presents some helpful words in this regard, in his article on integrating Buddhist meditation with peace education:

> The bowing to the Buddha statue does not necessarily have to mean the worship of a strange deity in the form of a statue. It can simply mean the acknowledgement of an ideal state of consciousness. Joseph Campbell once conveyed that bowing to the form of a deity was recognising the state of consciousness represented in it in one's own self [148].

In other words, God or the divine becomes a symbol of a greater understanding and the image of the deity becomes a marker to remind us of our practice (for those who hold the belief that imagery of the divine essence is malevolent, non-personified markers are imaginable). As a consequence we may understand the image not as the real thing but as a memory cue for the state of grace or consciousness that is being aspired to. *Bhakti* may also be understood as a concentration practice that may lead to the deeper inner meditation. According to the Patanjali yogic aphorism on concentration practices (1, 37):

> Or (by meditation on) the heart that has given up all attachment to sense-objects. Take some holy person, whom you revere, some saint whom you know to be perfectly non-attached, and think of his heart. That heart has become non-attached, and meditate on that heart; it will calm the mind [Vivekananda 1899, 1923, 2011, 155].

Slowly the practitioner imbibes the qualities of the chosen consciousness as represented by the deity as a memory cue. This agrees with the common folk knowledge that "you are what you think you are" yet there is experimental research showing the underlying mechanisms of remembrance. In the ancient yogic practice of *japa*, inner and outer remembrance is focused on the divine. This may be understood as a form of inner mental conditioning. Current modern research has investigated the effects of positive inner mental conditioning on physical wellness. Levy, Pilver, Chung and Slade (2014) examined whether positive age stereotypes, presented subliminally across multiple sessions in the community, would lead to improved outcomes. One hundred older individuals (age = 61–99 years, M = 81) were randomly assigned to an implicit-positive-age-stereotype-intervention group, an explicit-positive-age-stereotype-intervention group, a combined implicit- and explicit-positive-age-stereotype-intervention group, or a control group. Interventions occurred at four 1-week intervals. The implicit intervention strengthened positive age stereotypes, which strengthened positive self-perceptions of aging which, in turn, improved physical function. The improvement in these outcomes continued for 3 weeks after the last intervention session. Further, negative age stereotypes and negative self-perceptions of aging were weakened. For all outcomes, the implicit intervention's impact was greater than the explicit intervention's impact. The physical-function effect of the implicit intervention surpassed a previous study's 6-month-exercise-intervention's effect with participants of similar ages. It is interesting that implicit inner processes can have such a powerful effect upon our health and may help us to understand the possible mechanisms of Bhakti Yoga.

Jnana Yoga Pathway

This is the path of knowledge and is the intellectual path to Yoga. This involves the study of ancient teachings and using the mind to understand its own nature. In Jnana Yoga there are six qualities to be cultivated: (i) *sama* (control of mind), (ii) *dama* (control of the senses), (iii) *uparati* (renunciation of activities that are not duties), (iv) *titiksha* (endurance), (v) *shraddha* (faith), and (vi) *samadhana* (perfect concentration). This "mental" path requires high levels of discipline and awareness. In Jnana Yoga the goal is to investigate the intellect to study and penetrate it. Considered the most difficult form of Yoga, the *Jnana* path clears the mind to understand the mind. *Viveka* (right discernment) and *Vairagya* (detachment) lift the concealing veils of the mind and, through divesting oneself of the illusions of reality, the truth can be revealed.

Karma Yoga Pathway

Karma is a Sanskrit term derived from the root word *kri*, which means doing an activity, which in this context includes mental, physical and vocal activities (Singh and Singh 2012). This is the pathway of egoless service, which acts as a model for moral development. In this the human being carries out their daily duties as if they are in devoted and tender service. There is no cultivation of attachment or ego. It is a simple surrender to the duties that our roles and lives give us, without any attachment or ego. Mulla and Krishnan (2006) performed a content analysis of the *Bhagavad-gita* and identified Karma Yoga as: (i) performing an action without attachment, (ii) doing one's duty, and (iii) being neutral to opposites. The *Bhagavad-gita* (2010) describes the mental attitude that the Karma Yoga practitioner cultivates as

> He attaches nothing to the results of his action. Thus gain and loss resulting from his actions mean the same to him. He doesn't need a purpose therefore to motivate him into action. Therefore do your duty without any attachment to the fruits of your work, for only by acting without attachment, you will be able to realise God [3, 18/19, 180].

According to Singh and Singh (2012) Karma Yoga can also be defined as skill in performing action; equability of mind towards outcomes of actions; and a tool to eliminate a sense of attachment (*Bhagavad-gita*, 2, 48, 50, 51). Attachment, in this sense, is not beneficial attachment (for example attachment between children to caregivers) but attachment that leads to negative by-products, feelings of discrimination that become judgmental and/or reactionary feelings. Such equanimity (a feeling of balance and emotional regulation) potentially creates a humble, global attitude towards life and a compassionate way of relating to ones' own lifestyle and responsibilities. Current research on compassionate goal setting shows an association with positive outcomes such as improved social bonds, enhanced wellbeing, reduced feelings of loneliness, depression and anxiety (Crocker and Canevello 2008). Sprecher and Fehr (2005) found that compassionate love was associated positively with empathy, helpfulness, volunteerism, and social support. Likewise, Mulla and Krishnan (2014), in their study of 459 of employees in two large Indian organizations, showed that the Karma Yoga orientations of duty orientation, indifference to rewards and equanimity were positively correlated with moral sensitivity, moral motivation and moral character. However, Simon Brodbeck (2007) in his comparison of elite cricketers and peak performance as exemplified by *Bhagavad-gita*, draws out such further aspects of Karma Yoga as, "performative excellence, of lack of agency, and of losing oneself in each moment as it happens (where 'self' is, as previously defined, the conventional person who stands to gain or lose)" (792). Brodbeck (2007) gives a modern example from the sports field that assists our understanding of how Karma Yoga might express itself in a modern setting:

> A typical account might run as follows: "I saw the ball come off the bat, and the next thing I knew I was on the ground, it was in my hand, and I realised I had caught it." Here the sense of agency, and indeed the sense of self, is supplied only retrospectively, when the player has, as it were, "come to" (which sometimes happens only at the prompting of his exultant teammates). In the case of great catches the suspension of agency is rather brief, but a similar phenomenon is indicated by the idea that batsmen and bowlers may find themselves "in the zone" (that is, playing in an effortlessly sublime fashion), perhaps even for whole sessions of play at a time. This spatial metaphor, which implies that the player in question is somewhere completely different from the other players on the same pitch (he is, we might say, transported), carries with it an idea similar to the one we have seen in the Bhagavadgita [792].

In this we see the practical aspects of non-attachment alongside execution of duty in an excellent manner. Rastogi and Pati (2015) defined Karma Yoga as "A persistent positive state of mind that is characterized by *absorption* and *service consciousness*. Furthermore, the findings also suggest the importance of *sense control* and *equanimity* as the necessary prerequisites for individuals to practice Karma Yoga" (51).

This research project, while useful, misses the importance of the internal base, which nourishes the "persistent positive state of mind" of the Karma Yoga practitioner. Salzberg (1995) reminds us:

> A way to discover intimacy with ourselves and all of life is to live with integrity, basing our lives on a vision of compassionate nonharming. When we dedicate ourselves to actions that do not hurt ourselves or others, our lives become all of one piece, a "seamless garment" with nothing separate or disconnected in the spiritual reality we discover [cited in Brantmeier 2007, 137].

What is this "intimacy with ourselves and all of life" that she suggests we can discover through the Karmic Yoga practice of service and non-harming? Perhaps it is simply the integration and unity with the "forceless force" of love (Ram Chandra 1991) alongside the awareness and experience of deep connection with all living beings.

Yogic Psychology

Yogic psychology, put simply, teaches that the human being wishes to be happy but is unable to achieve this while they have desire and attachment to objects. The material world of objects is impermanent and constantly changing. Therefore any joy so derived is followed by feelings of loss, change and misery. The three kinds of *duhkha* (suffering) are those triggered by the individual's *self-caused* internal atmosphere within the body; those instigated by natural and extra-organic causes, *adi bhautika* (agents outside of the body); and those initiated by supra-natural and extra-organic causes, *adi dairika* (unseen energies).

One way for human beings to be free of this cycle is to regulate the mind and reach the stage where the mind is no longer unruly (Prasada 1912; Dasgupta 1989; Prabhavananda 2012). From this state human beings have the possibility of realizing their true nature, which is said to be pure consciousness (Prasada 1912). The practices that lead to this state of pure consciousness have both an outward (*bhahiranga*) and an inward (*antaranga*) nature. The outward practices strengthen the systems in the body and the inward practices purify the mind. Both groups of practices are intertwined and interconnected. The outcomes of such regular and systematic practice are documented for all eight aspects of practice and it is understood that each practice contribute to the efficacy of the others.

Srivastava (2010) identifies the Indian perspective of human nature according an awareness of consciousness:

> The essence of personality is something beyond body, life, mind and intellect. It is Atman, the self. Its chief attribute is consciousness. The self exists before, in and after the various states of consciousness: wakeful, dream and sleep. Denial of consciousness means denial of everything else. Hence, mind and self are not identical. The self is knower (kshetrajna), the seer (drasta), the witness (sakshi), and the immutable (kutastha). The composite

whole of chit and achit (consciousness and matter), kshetrajna and kshetra (knower and known), karta and karana (doer and its instrument) is the total personality called Jiva and Jivatman—the embodied self. Jiva (the individual), Purusha (the person), Samsari (the worldly person), Vijnanaghana/Vijnanatma, Prajna, Atma/Pratyagatma, Sariri, Karta, Bhokta, and Kshetrajna are synonymous [78].

Principles of Yogic Lifestyle

The principles of a yogic lifestyle are simple and involve being in tune with nature. Most contemplative traditions speak of the value of getting out of bed as the sun rises and Yoga does also. The relative stillness as the night merges into day and as all the creatures wake up is said to be a time of balance and conducive to experiencing balance and a peaceful consciousness. Practitioners are encouraged to craft a lifestyle that allows inward practices such as: concentration, meditation, cultivation of attitudes of remembrance, gratitude, devotion and awareness. Outer practices include: breathing to still the mind, devotional objects to prompt remembrance and attitudes of gratitude, physiological poses, a calming diet and other lifestyle observances such as cleansing practices and asceticism. The use of the word "craft" is deliberate in this context as it takes skill, creativity and flexibility to merge these inner and outer practices with modern digital/industrial lifestyles.

> JANINE: At the Sanskrit University in India we were taught to blend our modern lives and technology with traditional Yogic practices, leading to and maintaining our experience of peaceful community living. Perhaps this was the start of a yogic peace education as we learnt to entrain ourselves through simple daily practices. If we are sick we sleep. When we are well we start the weekdays like this.
>
> In the morning we woke early to the sound of Sanskrit slokas being chanted melodically and broadcast through the University outside speaker system—the volume soft. Thus woken we would get out of our beds, have a glass of water and walk along the path amongst trees to the Yoga mandiram (studio temple). The males went into the ground floor Yoga studio on the right, the girls into the studio on the left. Our teacher would be cross-legged on a slightly raised platform calmly waiting for us. A slight smile, tension free dressed in white. We arrived as we woke mostly on time but not exactly. There was no negativity if someone arrived very late; just a quiet joining in. We were dressed in our ordinary day clothes: hair up, kohl around our eyes and bindis in place. Jewellery removed for the asana practice. We use our scarfs to keep our clothing discrete during the inversion

Part II: Yogic Science

poses. Interesting to not need special Yoga clothes or equipment. We begin by sitting in padmasana one meditation pose. A shared chanted Sanskrit song-prayer. We follow with simple breathing practices designed to open both nasal practices. I am surprised that one side is blocked as I have always breathed easily. Over a few months both sides open and balance. We stand and together to the asana sequence that salutes the sun. It makes sense as the sun is rising and we are already calm and feeling good. We don't move as a group. We go at our own pace according to the length and rhythm of our own in and out breathing. At the end we all go into shavasana. Once we have all returned to this pose we move into the next sequence of asanas. As we each finish a sequence we lie down on the ground. Once we have all had rest time we start the next sequence of poses together. No competition, no stress. We are absorbed in our own quiet process. Our breathing. The poses improve over time, almost as an add-on. Not the goal. I am deeply relaxed as I move. It's almost a gentle dance. Once we have completed the final asana we sit together in meditation. We follow with a short Sanskrit prayer of devotion-thanks-gratitude. Walking back for breakfast the girls collect flowers that have fallen on the ground. The air is fragrant. We are calm and aware. The flowers will be used for puja as some of the girls also follow the religious Hindu devotional practices.

KATERINA: My yogic lifestyle could not be more different. I was at my most "yogic" when I was studying as a fulltime grad student, working at the YMCA and teaching 10–12 Yoga Classes a week. My week was filled with ethical and dietary restraints that I hoped would permit my yogic instrument (body-mind-spirit) to endure being the vessel of everybody else's wellness while somewhat managing my own. A frequently typical day for me: I rose at 6:00 am to try to manage one cup of coffee before driving through town and parking before the meters activated (you can't get a parking ticket before 9:00 in my town) to teach "rise 'n' shine" Power Yoga at 7:00 am at the Y (rule #1: I could not eat more than 2 hours before teaching or drink one hour before teaching or I would have to run to the bathroom or be sluggish or burp from digestion). Then after my first class I would bust across town to the 90 minute free parking zone across the bridge (rule #2: parking costs money and parking tickets are not affordable for grad students so at all costs park for free or ride your bike) and sprint to one of the Yoga studio's I taught at (there were four) and teach the 9–10:30 Hatha Yoga class. I worked at the Y at 11:00 so I would run back to my car, grab a bad muffin and another cup of coffee on the way and study for 15 minutes in clothes I had already taught two classes in before putting on my uniform at the Y. From 11:00–4:00 I would work at the Y giving out squash racquet's or locker keys at the front desk and sometimes be called upon to teach a gentle flow class at 1:00 (if the teacher was a no-show) that is why I never ate until my 15 minute break at 1:30 (government mandated) in case I had to run upstairs to the Y Yoga studio and teach. I would have just enough time during my 15-minute break to go get another bad muffin coffee and make it until my next class at 4:30. From then until 5:50 I taught my favorite class of the day at my favorite Yoga studio and lo and behold ... while showing up to sign in for my class learned that the very popular 6:00–7:20 teacher was called in to the hospital to work so "could I also sub his class." The answer was always ... yes. Tuition, rent, food, bad muffins, gas ... it all costs money. I was very grateful for my classes and happy to sub for others but the transactions of teaching and living and studying and constantly moving meant the only time my body wasn't moving or getting into position to move was during the tune in. That was my little oasis.

Conclusions

Yogic Science is a holistic discipline comprised of eight key practices. These practices affect the physiology, psychology and behavior of individuals and the communities in which they belong. The human being who achieves Yoga experiences a restraining of "mind-stuff" from taking various forms such as preoccupied thought, and is able to achieve clarity, calmness and inner stillness. From this comes the capability to master his or her outer behaviors and move into a consciousness of connection with others. In this the individual becomes a potential embodiment of peace, capable of crafting a lifestyle based upon inner consciousness, rather than dogma and restrictions. As Joyce (2015) states: "A peace, which happens naturally because we no longer experience our self-identity as isolated from the 'Other,' who is each other" (240).

FOUR

Yoga and Life Nourishment

He toi whakairo
He mana tangata
Where there is artistic excellence
There is human dignity.

Introduction

Perhaps an indigenous Māori proverb seems an unusual way to begin our next conversation about the life nourishing qualities of Yoga but we would like you to consider Yoga and your potential engagement as a Yogic peace educator as an art—and expression of creativity. It is an art in the sense that each of us has the capability to use our imaginations to entrain our nervous system in peaceful ways but it is also a science as Yoga describes practices that lead our neuro-psychobiological systems towards inner and outer balance. It is from this "art-science" balance that we ourselves become instruments of creative change. Peacebuilding, generally speaking, is an intervention: an action that can lead to change. In this way, we consider Yogic Peace Education as a form of Yogic peacebuilding. The art and science of Yogic peacebuilding facilitate and create change that leads Yogic peace educators to elicit inner dignity in all that we do.

Ahimsa

We recall from previous chapters that *ahimsa* was defined as the practice of non-harming and described as, "not injuring others by thought, word or deed" (Vivekânanda 1899, 295). It is one (and the first listed) of the individual restraints or capacities to be developed within a practitioner of Yogic Science. It refers to an "aspirant's attitude towards the outer world and towards himself, in short, to ethics and morality in the widest sense of those terms" (Wood 1959, 37). At its strictest manifestation, *ahimsa* is the dictate to not kill or be violent towards others, including all forms of animal, plant and mineral life. In this chapter we recognize that the practice of complete external *ahimsa* is impossible to achieve in the global interconnected, geo-political-economic sphere that we inhabit. However, *it is possible* for most human beings to aspire to a life-caring or a life-nourishing practice; *it is possible* to stop acts of direct violence; and *it is also possible* for individuals to embody in their own subtle mind field the quality of *ahimsa*. It is these attitudes that we suggest promote a natural life-nourishing stance.

In this chapter we will explore the Systems Network Model of Yoga for Optimizing Self-Regulation (Gard, Noggle, Park, Vago and Wilson 2014) to understand the physiological mechanisms underlying a life-nourishing rendition of *ahimsa*. We will discuss the possible psychological and relational effects of a life nourishing perspective and touch on the classical understandings of the subtle energetic[1] effects of *ahimsa*.

The Art and Science of *Ahimsa*

While we have asked you to consider Yoga as an art, counterintuitively we also understand it as a science—a practical activity that leads to new information. As previously identified, Yogic Science is an integrated practice and includes all eight practices of Patanjali's codification system. In other words, each practice strengthens and subtly influences the other. All the practices of *yama*/observance combine to purify the inner mind and outer body of the practitioner:

> The transactions of life are between the real man (purusha) or Self (ātmā) and the world, but there are two instruments in between, as it were—the mind as inner instrument and the body as outer instrument. These two tools—or perhaps we should call them kits, as they are both quite complex—have to be put into good order and kept in good order as part of the regular system of conditioning [Wood 1959, 37].

Sattvification includes the refinement of consciousness, a process that takes time and involves both mental and behavioral conditioning.

Simply put *sattvification* is a process of sensory-motor integration (proprioceptive, cardiovascular, pulmonary, musculoskeletal, vestibular and sensory) alongside conditioning of low and high level brain networks (influenced by ethics, breath control, meditation and sustained postures) (Gard et al. 2014). This in turn leads to an inhibition within the person of: (i) negative appraisal, (ii) emotional reactivity, (iii) rumination, (iv) inflammation, (v) muscle tension and pain, and (vii) vasopulmonary constriction. The output of regular Yogic conditioning upon these systems is seen externally as: (i) pro-social and ethical behavior, (ii) psychological and physical wellbeing, and (iii) musculoskeletal strengthening (Gard et al. 2014). It is these processes that have been described classically according to religious or ethical experience, or as the yogic purification of consciousness: "These ethical and moral heights which are thus taught as the very beginning of the Yoga path are announced not merely as leading to inward benefit. Their effects are stated to permeate the external living also" (Wood 1959, 45).

In these words, we can see that the practice of *yama*/restraint is a preparation for the development of a deeper integration of one's inner consciousness. The diligent Yoga practitioner has the possibility of developing mental resilience and becomes less likely to be overtaken by negative thoughts, attachment to outer objects, cravings, and rumination. This psychological development is in itself potentially life nourishing; for example, less outer attachment and cravings for objects may show itself in greedlessness or in tolerant relational styles. In addition to neuro-psychobiological effects, Yogic practitioners are encouraged to be aware of themselves as spiritual and energetic beings—not solely corporeal matter made of cells, flesh and bone.

Here Yogic Science proposes an additional two bodies or levels of human existence—the causal (spiritual or karmic) sphere and the energetic (astral, psychic, *pranic*) sphere—planes or "bodies" of existence that have profound effects on our physical, emotional, psychological and mental being (see Figure 3).

Yoga Anatomy and *Ahimsa*

Yogic Science differs from Western science conceptually and we are hindered in our understanding of the effects of *ahimsa* on the physical and energetic body by words that hold similar but not identical

FIGURE 3
The Three Bodies

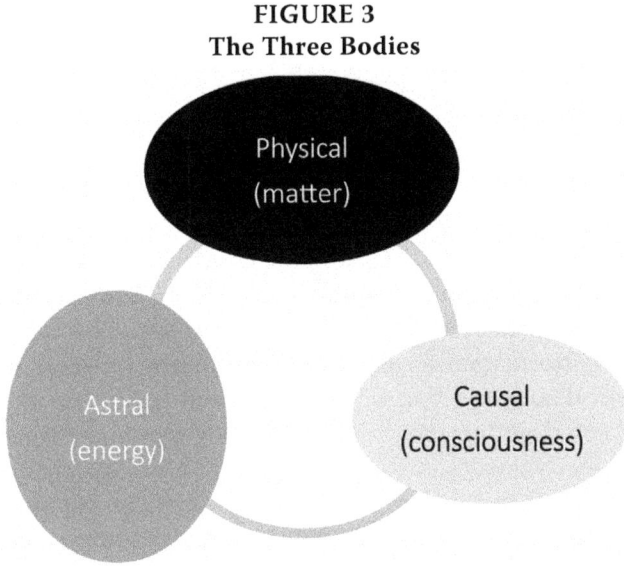

meanings that suggest immanent though imprecise categorizations (as we have already seen in this simple exploration of the energetic field). Western considerations separate the body, for example, into the muscular, the skeletal, the endocrinal and the neurological systems, and each segment of the human physical existence here refers to an agreed upon collection of matter—the nervous system is not a part of the skeletal system, etc. But to understand the conceptualizations of *Yoga*, it is necessary to adopt an alternative understanding of the human instrument as an organism that exists in a both a physical sense and an energetic sense. This means that the tissues of our bodies do not bind our existence nor do we only have a perceptible impact on our individual selves.

According to Yogic Science, past experiences of *ahimsa* at a *causal* level created subtle impressions housed in an inner seed or soul that is comprised of impressions accumulated over many lifetimes (*karma*). The experience of *ahimsa* at the *energetic* level manifests, in the present, in our mental, intellectual and physical wellbeing. It is very difficult to describe the effects of *ahimsa* on the energetic system without a prior understanding of Yoga Anatomy. The Anatomy of Yoga[2] recognizes that each of us have, not one but three (overlapping) bodies—the physical body (made of food), the causal body (containing the karmic seed or soul) and the energetic body (comprised of the mind, the intellect and the *Pranic* sheath). Dispensing with the causal (spiritual body) as that is formed by past impressions, we can now examine the energetic and physical bodies and the effects of *ahimsa*.

Yogic Science considers the *citta* as an electromagnetic field—existing in both the energetic *and* physical bodies—that is naturally tuned to life nourishing considerations in response to stimuli received by the sensory-motor system. Although we tend to think of our senses as *physical* or housed within our physicality, Yogic Science categorizes the senses as existing as both *physical* and *energetic*. This is a key conceptual transformation for most of us—it means we sense with our non-physical body and that we are always and continually sensing as opposed to feeling "sensations" that are momentary and responsive to taste, touch, temperature, etc. Significantly, for our understanding of how we respond to stimulation, the natural, spontaneous state of the *citta* is life nourishing. This life nourishing default setting means that, according to Yogic Science, our neuro-psychobiological system naturally experiences non-animosity towards the external world as brought to us through our sensory-motor systems. Through yogic discipline we can increase our life nourishing "setting." Importantly, through Yogic Science we not only cease being antagonistic to things we feel, we stop being hostile to things we can only imagine.

The Sanskrit word *manas* translates in the English language as "mind." Our minds receive information from our sensory-motor systems and this information impacts directly upon our physical and energetic bodies. As our *manas* (mind) perceives information from the senses, it is incorporated into our energetic body. This system is comprised of *chakras* (center of vital energy) and *nadis*, subtle and invisible energetic pathways and vortices analogous to the neurological system in Western medicine or the meridian system of Traditional Chinese Medicine (TCM). Western (neurology) and Eastern (Yoga, TCM) energy systems are largely invisible to the naked eye although some dedicated expert observers can see evidence of these systems through personal or scientific tools of perception.

CHAKRAS

Yogic science conceptualizes that *prana* (life energy) comprises and manifests a vital sheath, or strata, of energy that surrounds and inhabits the human body (around, within and of you). This configuration houses the *chakra* system (a system where pranic energy flows along one's energetic pathways) and is considered fundamental to wellbeing. Physically, *pranic* energy travels along energy pathways (*nadis*) converging to a vertical column called the *sushumna*.

The base of the *sushumna* rests on the perineum and travels upwards to the crown of the head. The feminine aspect of *pranic* energy travels along the left, calming, lunar side of the body and is called the *ida*. The masculine aspect of pranic energy travels along the right, energizing, solar side of the body and is called the *pingala*. Seven energy centers exist along the line of the *sushumna* where the *ida* and *pingala* intertwine. These centers are called *chakras*, literally, wheels of light. And, whereas the physical body has organs of operation (pancreas or heart for example) and systems of vitality (the circulatory system for instance) the *chakras* are the organs of the energetic body, picking up vibrations, transforming and distributing energy.

In Yogic Science there are ways of targeting or focusing on our personal wellbeing using Chakra Yoga, Yoga designed to balance the energetic system and release blocked or overactive chakras. Chakra Yoga is practiced similarly to other therapeutic modalities requiring expertise, experience and sensitivity (attributes of the *chakras* such as colors associated with each energy vortex or the qualities of physical or mental processes on each one could fill a whole book and we encourage interested readers to delve further into this modality of understanding). While an exhaustive exploration of the remedial and therapeutic practices of Chakra Yoga are beyond the scope of this book interested readers can peruse the following information to imagine how each of these vital energy vortices impacts our wellbeing.

1. ***Muladhara*** (translated: root, support)
   Location: Pelvic Floor, Perineum
   ***Bija* Seed Sound:** Lam (pronounced *lum*)
   Sense: Smell (Earth creates smell)
   Element: Earth
   Food: Proteins
   Domain: Basic Needs-survival, scarcity, trust
   Season: Winter
   Yoga Path: Hatha Yoga

Life Stage: Baby
Emotion: Stillness
Poses: Squat, Mountain, Standing Squat, Warriors

2. *Svadisthana* (translated: sweetness)
    Location: Pelvic Basin, Lower Belly
    ***Bija* Seed Sound:** Vam (pronounced *vum*)
    Sense: Taste (Water enables taste)
    Element: Water
    Food: Liquids
    Domain: Passions, Creativity, desire, lust
    Season: Spring
    Yoga Path: Tantra Yoga
    Life Stage: Puberty
    Emotion: Tears
    Poses: bow, goddess pose, hip circles, knee down twist, half moon, dancer

3. *Manipura* (translated: lustrous jewel, filled with jewels)
    Location: Solar Plexus
    ***Bija* Seed Sound:** Ram (pronounced *rum*)
    Sense: Sight (Fire illuminates)
    Domain: power
    Element: Fire
    Food: Starches
    Season: Summer
    Yoga Path: Karma Yoga
    Life Stage: Young adult, work
    Emotion: Laughter, anger, joy
    Poses: woodchopper, sun salutations, upward boat, incline

4. *Anahata* (translated: unstruck sound)
    Location: Heart
    ***Bija* Seed Sound:** Yam (pronounced *yum*)
    Sense: touch (air enables touch) touch food, people, self with love
    Domain: love
    Element: air
    Food: vegetables
    Season: Fall

Four. Yoga and Life Nourishment

    Yoga Path: Bakti Yoga, unconditional devotion
    Life Stage: Family
    Emotion: compassion, unconditional love, selfless service
    Poses: birds: eagle, crow, Camel, star gazer, triangle, cow face, cobra

5. *Vishuddhi* (translated: purification)
    Location: Neck
    ***Bija* Seed Sound:** Ham (pronounced *hum*)
    Sense: sound (space allows sound to travel)
    Domain: communication
    Element: ether
    Food: Fruits
    Yoga Path: Mantra Yoga
    Life Stage: after menopause, andropause
    Emotion: connection, communication, expression
    Poses: shoulder stand, plow, fish, neck rolls, lion, rabbit

6. *Ajna* (translated: to perceive)
    Location: third eye
    ***Bija* Seed Sound:** ksham (also uw in some traditions)
    Color: Violet (indigo)
    Sense: Inner Intuition
    Domain: awareness and wisdom
    Food: Mind-altering substances
    Yoga Path: Yantra *Yoga*
    Life Stage: wise years
    Emotion: Dreaming
    Poses: Yoga mudra, eye Yoga

7. *Sahasrara* (translated: thousand fold)
    Location: crown of the head
    ***Bija* Seed Sound:** Aum (also silence in some traditions)
    Domain: spirituality
    Element: thought- beyond the elements
    Food: fasting
    Yoga Path: Jnana Yoga
    Life Stage: withdrawal from society
    Emotion: Bliss
    Poses: Lotus, headstand

The seven centers in the energetic system are concerned with receiving sensory information and are located in the following areas: (i) base of the spine, (ii) at the nexus of the sacral and lumbar spine, (iii) solar plexus, (iv) sternum, (v) throat, (vi) third eye (between and slightly upwards from the eyebrows), and (vii) top of the head (Feuerstein 2001) (see Figure 4).

It is these centers that are purified by the eight stages (ash-tang) of Patanjali's Yoga. It is here, in these subtle aspects of the human system (in the Astral Body) that *ahimsa* and other Yogic practices transform us. Whicher (1998) describes it thusly: "Through a process termed the sattvification (purifying) of consciousness, the mental processes of the yogin are remolded, reshaped and restructured leading to a transformation of the mind and its functioning" (85).

There has been a great deal of investigation done on this area of human functioning by *yogins*. Many *yogins* have written detailed accounts of their practices and their resultant changes in consciousness. By modern research standards, these data would be seen in the category of case reports and can be considered an excellent base for more rigorous testing. The current capacity of neuro imaging has allowed verification of what has been described philosophically and/or experientially by dedicated *yogins*.

FIGURE 4
Charka Energy Centers, Names and Locations

Chakra	Name	Location
7	*Sahasra*	Crown
6	*Ajna*	3rd Eye
5	*Vishuddi*	Throat
4	*Anahata*	Sternum
3	*Manipura*	Solar Plexus
2	*Svadisthana*	Sacrum
1	*Mooladhara*	Coccyx

In 2014 Fox et al. reviewed 123 brain morphology differences (form, shape or structure) from 21 neuroimaging studies, with three hundred participants. They found eight functional capabilities consistently altered in meditators: meta-awareness; exteroceptive and interoceptive body awareness; memory consolidation and reconsolidation; self and emotion regulation; and inner neurological communication (48). Marchand's (2014) meta-analysis on mindfulness meditation cited studies, which identify 16 brain regions subject to mindfulness related changes. He concluded that this form of meditation affected the structure of the medial cortex, associated default mode network and the basal ganglia (Marchand 2014, 471) demonstrating "compelling evidence that mindfulness impacts the function [of the brain]" (476).

Compassion meditation, from the Tibetan tradition, by expert practitioners (over 10,000 hours) shows activation of the brain in the motor region. The motor region is simply the area of the brain responsible for the planning, control and execution of voluntary movement. Authors Back, Bauer-Wu, Rushton and Halifax (2009) wondered whether compassion meditation done in this way created a state of readiness to act. They demonstrated neural integration, as evidenced by high-amplitude gamma-band oscillation, in experienced meditation practitioners, suggestive of the beneficial effects of contemplative practice on cognitive and affective functioning (Back et al. 2009). Meditation teacher Osho Rajneesh helps us to understand the role of meditation: "We have to save ourselves from our own minds. This mind was created for a certain reason: to save us from the animals. For centuries we were in danger; now we are in danger from our own destructive weapons" (1988, 26).

Rajneesh reminds us that the emotion of fear in the human being is the underlying motivation for attitudes and behaviors of greed, violence and theft. To go beyond this cognitive mind, we may need to understand *manas*. *Manas* and the influence of *ahimsa* upon *manas* remain a fertile area for future investigation.

AHIMSA AS A NATURAL PROCESS

Traditionally, the knowledge of Yogic Science was transmitted from teacher to student. Teacher and student lived closely together in family and community. It was an unspoken process, subtler than psychological processes of modeling or cognitive processes of speaking/listening. In some way, the transferal of the knowledge of *ahimsa* was a natural attunement from the teacher's heart or *manas*, to the *manas* of the student; one person to another—one heart-mind to another.

Currently, many Western Yoga practitioners are entering this science through the pathway of rehabilitation or maintenance for the physical or psychological needs of the body. Fitness classes and short courses on meditation and mindfulness are taking the place of deep attunement with the teacher. Traditionally, *ahimsa* manifests externally on the personality as a growing conscious sensitivity and identification of what constitutes violence. The individual begins to develop a sense of unity with the outer world and this connectivity may lead to questions about the limits of external *ahimsa*. Many questions arise at this point. Is it an act of violence to over consume and contribute to environmental degradation and destructive climate change? Is it okay to kill for food? Is it okay to use one's willpower to achieve excellence in a system designed to impose explicit and implicit inequality? There are no absolute right answers to these questions and others like them but answers accumulate as a process of awareness and congruence with one's own changing consciousness. In this way Yogic Science does not prescribe rules about what one should or should not believe. One does not impose *ahimsa* on oneself; as one's heart opens it becomes natural to not want to hurt another. This is the step into a life nourishing practice. It starts with gross (physical) acts and later begins to include subtle acts of nonviolence in the use of words and in the quality of one's thoughts. Thought includes the practice of both active thinking and automated thinking.

> Knowing is not thinking. Knowing begins when thinking ceases having finished its work. Every new knowing is a joy, for it is a new experience of unity—something perfectly attuned and non-conflicting in Nature has conveyed its lesson, nay, has entered and enriched the being of the consciousness, just as edibles and air enter the body and become part of it [Wood 1959, 60].

It is this knowing that can be described as natural; requiring no thought, willpower, or determination. It is outside of the purely cognitive or higher levels of brain function. It is a deep integration of neural pathways and it leads to the right action, seemingly without much ruminative thought, or even any thought, in each circumstance. It is characterized by a deep inner joy or *santosha*. The inner condition of *santosha* is a natural condition of balance, which may be sensed in the equanimity and poise of the practitioner or the degree of balance and ease in their responsiveness to the outer environment.

Physiological Mechanisms of Yoga

Yoga creates optimal self-regulation seen physiologically, neurologically, behaviorally and psychologically. To understand the multifaceted interplay between Yoga practice and wellness Gard et al. compiled a Systems Networks Model (2014: 6) to illustrate the complex interrelationship of four aspects of Yoga practice (see Figure 5) and impacts on both high and low level brain networks and on sensory processes (see Figure 6). The authors argue that the neurological processes which allow self-regulation become more automatized and efficient over time and with sustained practice, require less effort to initiate when necessary and terminate when no longer needed (Gard et al. 2014, 770). The model is extremely complex but has been simplified in the following three images (for the full model we encourage readers to visit the original publication). To begin, we need to understand which yogic practices are considered the foundation of the model (see Figure 5).

As has already been mentioned, yogic practices include a variety of exercises—some internal and some external. Internal exercises

FIGURE 5
Four Yogic Practices from Gard et al. 2014

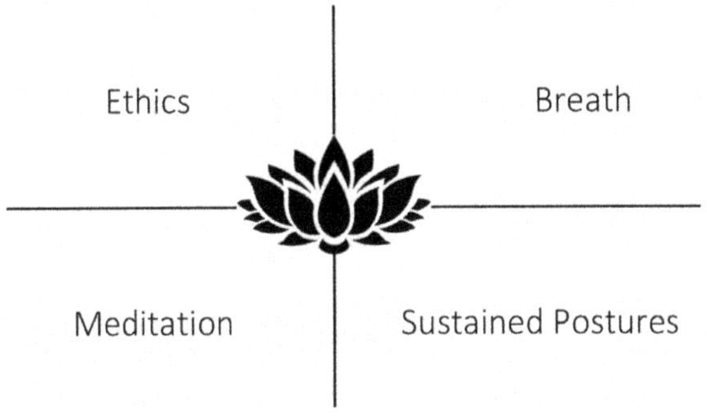

Ethics	Breath
Meditation	Sustained Postures

include the ethical observances and restraints (*yamas* and *niyamas*) as well as contemplative pursuits such as mental focusing (*dharana*) and meditation (*dhyana*). External exercises involve movement or breath (*pranayama*) or body (*asana*) or both (*Hatha Yoga*). Yogic Science tells us that these internal and external practices are each impactful on their own but when combined, compound wellness. Gard et al. (2014) observes these four yogic practices in their relation to both low-level and high-level brain networks (see Figure 6).

Yoga entrains the neuro-psychobiological system to function optimally and in this state it is natural for the human being to feel more relaxed, comfortable and resilient in response to outer stimuli. It may be natural for such a developed nervous system to feel blissful (*santosha*). It is useful to be explicit, and we consider that it has been difficult to render the qualities of these subtle inner conditions into the English language. *Santosha* is not a condition of euphoria or ecstasy. Euphoria and ecstasy are not considered optimal within Yoga as they may lead to damage within the human nervous system, particularly if such states continue for a long duration. The condition of *santosha* is experienced as a deep and natural state of balance and does no damage to the human instrument.

The processes of Yoga create a neuro-psychobiological system which experiences wellness, expresses ethical and prosocial behavior and has a strong musculoskeletal structure. Although a yogic peacebuilder is more than a neuro-psychobiological system (we are not simply human instruments), an optimally functioning system is an excellent place to begin. When we personally experience wellness and acquire physical, emotional, psychological and mental resilience, we have much more to offer one another. We have the capability to develop a clear minded, inner awareness of our own habitual reactions; we have an opportunity to appreciate information we receive from the outside world without hostility; and we have the capability to reprogram ourselves away from thoughts, words and deeds that are violent.

Life Nourishing *Ahimsa*

In book II, sutra 35 of Patanjali's *Yoga Sutras*, the first *yama*/observance, *ahimsa* (nonviolence) is described: "*ahimsâ pratisthayam tat samnidhau vaira tyagah*/in the presence of one firmly established in

FIGURE 6
Systems Network Model of Yoga

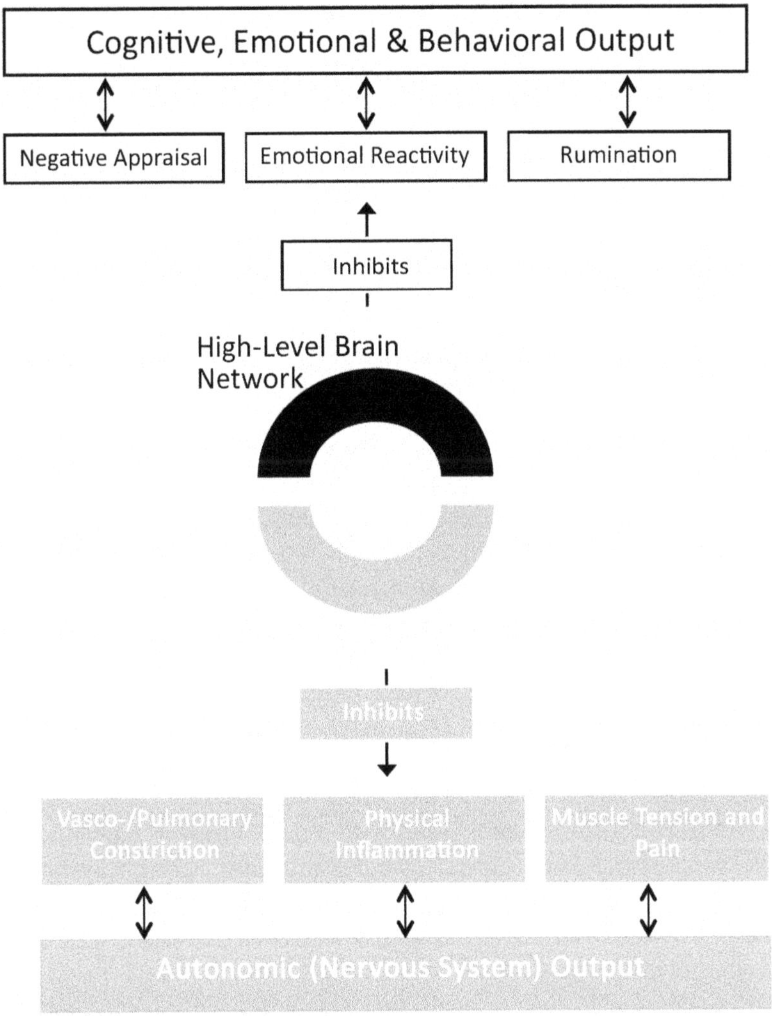

```
┌─────────────────────────────────────────────────┐
│   Cognitive, Emotional & Behavioral Output      │
└─────────────────────────────────────────────────┘
        ↕              ↕              ↕
┌──────────────┐ ┌──────────────────┐ ┌────────────┐
│Negative      │ │Emotional         │ │Rumination  │
│Appraisal     │ │Reactivity        │ │            │
└──────────────┘ └──────────────────┘ └────────────┘
                         ↑
                  ┌─────────────┐
                  │  Inhibits   │
                  └─────────────┘

          High-Level Brain
          Network

                  ┌─────────────┐
                  │  Inhibits   │
                  └─────────────┘
                         ↓
┌──────────────┐ ┌──────────────────┐ ┌────────────────┐
│Vasco-/Pulmo- │ │Physical          │ │Muscle Tension  │
│nary          │ │Inflammation      │ │and Pain        │
│Constriction  │ │                  │ │                │
└──────────────┘ └──────────────────┘ └────────────────┘
        ↕              ↕                     ↕
┌─────────────────────────────────────────────────┐
│     Autonomic (Nervous System) Output           │
└─────────────────────────────────────────────────┘
```

nonviolence, all hostilities cease" (Weiss 2006, 25). This is a powerful statement and one that is borne out anecdotally when people share their experience of being with those who have mastered themselves in such a way:

> When the vow of *ahimsâ* is established in someone, all enmity will cease in his or her presence because of the harmonious vibrations the person

emits. If two people who have enmity come to such a person, they will cease their hostilities in the presence of this person [Weiss 2006, 1].

Sahaj Marg Master Sri Babuji describes that the highest service a human being can offer to one another is to become someone whose mere presence creates an unbounded peace that permeates everywhere, throughout the atmosphere and throughout human interactions (Ram Chandra 1991). He writes:

> World peace is the crying need of the day and those at the top are trying hard to bring it about. But the means adopted for the purpose do not so far seem to promise fruitful results. The efforts for the establishment of world peace do not seem to be very effective only for the reason that they are merely external, touching only the fringes of the problem. As a matter of fact world peace can never be possible unless we take into account the inner state of the individual mind. World peace is directly related with individual peace, for which the individual mind is to be brought up to the required level [Ram Chandra 1991, 87].

This is the fundamental consideration in Yoga—that there is an abiding interconnectivity between peace within individuals and peace in the surrounding world. If world peace is an authentic objective, methods are required which can stimulate peacefulness. Sri Babuji relates that as world peace relates to individual peace it is essential to "find out means for developing within each individual a state of peace and contentment [so that] ... all that we have to do for the attainment of world peace is to mold the mental tendencies of the people individually ... [through a] proper regulation of the mind so as to introduce into it a state of moderation" (cited in Ram Chandra 1991, 87).

Yogic scientist Sivananda stated that nonviolence is a most effective master-method to counteract and eradicate completely the brutal, cruel traits of the individual (Suneetha 2013). The capacity to practice either *yama*/restraint or *ahimsa* continuously is unusual, as the following words acknowledge:

> Patanjali acknowledges that only those very rare beings in all the worlds (*sarvabhaumah*) who have taken a "great vow" (*mahavratam*) are able to practice all five *yamas* without interruption (*vicchinna*), while the rest of us must adapt these guidelines to our current occupation (*jati*), the place we live (*desa*), time of day, month, or year (*kala*), or circumstance (*samaya*). For example, if one who made his living (*jati*) fishing adhered firmly to the yamas ... he would not be able to practice *ahimsâ* unless he gave up his occupation, and hence harmed his family or himself by not being able to provide. Similarly, in the place where you live (*desa*), fresh

vegetables may not be available year-round, and it may be better for your health to supplement your diet with meat [Holcombe 2015, 32].

According to these voices the practice of *yama*/restraint for ordinary Yoga aspirants involves discretion and common sense. Chandrasekaran (2012) reminds us that *ahimsa* is not merely the absence of violence; it is also the presence of qualities, such as kindness and consideration. At a much deeper level it is the presence of non-animosity towards all forms of life. Which leads to further queries: what does the presence of non-animosity towards all forms of life mean? What would it mean to be embodied in a neuro-psychobiological system that was integrated in this way? What would it feel like? How would we be different from our current consciousness? What is our current state of consciousness? Do we seek peace; speak peace; action peace; yet from an inner state of animosity, judgment and force? What if we all pause and perhaps observe our own levels of non-animosity—as a process of awareness and observation and without any judgment. Can you observe the quality of your own *manas* (mind)? Try. What are your automatic reactions towards different political or religious beliefs? Think of a different way of living, loving or learning—what do you encounter in your mind? Or something less imaginary, perhaps—how do you react to physical discomfort—to feelings of being cold or hot, itchy or uncomfortable? It is very useful to observe our natural responses to our environments or discern our mental tendencies. Once we have spent some time investigating our usual (automatic) responses to stimuli we can consider reprogramming ourselves.

For example: one can begin the day by intending that the presence of non-animosity flow from your heart to others. When your brain or body reacts to certain words, ideas, behaviors that are outside of you, allow yourself to relax. Observe and practice sincerely for a gradually longer period of time. In this way we observe the science of ourselves and practice the art of evolving an inner human dignity.

Planning for Change

According to Yogic Science, the life force flows through all animate and inanimate objects. We perceive this according to the acuity of our own sensory apparatus. Over time we have all developed and been conditioned towards both aversion and attraction, and towards certain ideas and objects. Perhaps we can acknowledge that the development of a natural *ahimsa* towards all forms that contain life force is challenging and perhaps naïve.

The underlying principle of nonviolence is the unity of body, mind, and spirit, a "heart unity" (Nagler 2004) of self and others in the interconnectedness of life. The notion of heart unity refers to human connections beneath differences. Unity, the ultimate goal of Yoga, is based upon the far-reaching internal changes developed from the natural achievement of *ahimsa*: "The meaning of unity ... implies entire non-antagonism towards the world, and entire non-conflict within the yogi's own mind" (Wood 1959, 19).

The teaching of *ahimsa* is multifactorial and at its best is a direct non-spoken transmission of knowledge between the heart of the teacher and student. This resonates with thoughts about teaching nonviolence—the foundational goal of peace education. "The teacher's work on herself to achieve internal and interpersonal unity is essential to practicing a pedagogy of nonviolence for students to achieve inner peace" (Bolliger and Wang 2013, 113).

In this *ahimsa* is a quality of the heart-mind—a quantum field expressed through the instrument of mind and body. In this sense it is natural rather than occurring through a focus of concentration or behavior—something *that is*, not something *that is done*.

Spreading the Sphere

The interconnectivity of life means no person is an "energetic" island and that an essential separation (separate-ness) between humans (and all life) is false. Brantmeier and Lin (2008) remind us that, "Inner and outer peace are interdependent dimensions of the human experience. *Being* in peace and *doing* peace are united" (4).

> An understanding of the fundamental and radical interconnectedness of all life must serve as a rock bottom foundation for peace education endeavors. Without this sense of unity, of commonality, of collective humanity or of collective planetary coexistence, the value of the "other" life forms lessens and acts of violence against the "other" are justified, human normative structures prioritise life forms and hierarchies are created to justify the domination, oppression, or killing of the "other" based on positions of privilege established in those hierarchies [Brantmeier and Lin 2008, 152].

Four. Yoga and Life Nourishment

From the yogic perspective "being," "doing," "feeling" or "remembering" can create the inner changes of neuro-psychobiological and spiritual integration, such that peace becomes a natural expression of those humans devoted to transformative processes. Furthermore, according to Vivekânanda, an integrated mind receives intuitive knowledge without effort via inspirational flashes that are for the good of the world, perfectly unselfish and do not contradict reason (1923).

LIFE NOURISHMENT AS UNITY

Peace education within Yogic Science begins with the development of the capacity for felt unity. It is developed in the Yogic tradition through a range of steps culminating in meditation. Like Buddhism, mindful acceptance is a state of being that develops along the way. This does not lead to lethargy in action; rather it is expressed in the development of immense focus, responsiveness and the capacity to manage emotions and thoughts in a purposeful way. According to Kabat-Zinn (1994), mindfulness begins with the capacity to pay attention, "paying attention in a particular way: on purpose, in the present moment, and non-judgmentally" (4). *On purpose* refers to the capacity to choose to move into your experience in a present moment and non-evaluative state, and *the capacity to accept* includes an integration of qualities such as willingness, openness, compassion, kindness and playfulness (Eifert and Forsyth 2008).

CALM IN THE STORM

As one's capacity to view thoughts and feelings as a mental projection grows, one experiences the development of a soft, impartial inner observer. It is this capacity that is useful when living in conflictual environments and in difficult situations. The combination of acceptance, awareness and the soft inner observer lead to an opportunity for transformation regardless of circumstances. As George H. Eifert and John P. Forsyth share in *The Mindfulness and Acceptance Workbook for Anxiety*:

> If you can feel, and can stay with, the energy in your body- neither acting on it nor suppressing it—you can harness it in the service of actions that

move you forward toward achieving your valued goals. The raw energy of anxiety is fuel. You get to choose to use that fuel for you or against you [2008, 195].

In Yoga this raw energy is focused through the awareness of unity and interconnectedness with all manifestations of the life force. Practitioners describe a natural sensitivity towards other human beings and forms of life. Over time they embody a consciousness that is connected and unified in a profound and subtle way. In this experience the mind turns from non-harming towards life caring; from individual to collective; towards "other as each other" (Joyce, 2015). Again the words of Brantmeier (2007) are useful: "Understanding the essential unity of all life provides the necessary foundation for nonviolence in the world because violence against the 'other' is then understood as violence against the 'self'" (154). The oppositional stance of combatants, competitors or opponents becomes illusionary here, as any act against "another" becomes an action against "me." This unitary logic defies customary dualistic perceptions that imagine separate-ness between humans and the natural world, and between humans and other humans. What Brantmeier entreats is a new kind of warrior—one whose actions are enriched by this realization.

> We need extremists who are not against anything.... Right now, we are creating extremists who are always against somebody. The terrorists, for example, are causing havoc on this planet. But there is a certain dimension to them, which is very valuable. Terrorists are willing to die for what they hold as valuable.... Suppose they had no enemy. Suppose you had no enemy, you were incapable of making an enemy, but you were an extremist. You would be a fantastic, intense human being [2007, 154].

Conclusions

In this chapter we have discussed the notion of *ahimsa* as a process of developing a life nourishing perspective. We have understood such a perspective as coming from a self-regulated neuro-psychobiological system (Gard et al. 2014). We have discussed the possible psychological and relational effects of a life nourishing perspective. We have also identified components for developing and entraining oneself as a presence of *ahimsa*.

While we have presented one subset of Yoga's "comprehensive skillset," it is sensible to remember that it is one aspect of an interconnected series of practices that have deep effect on a multitude of neuropsychobiological processes. In the next chapter we turn to the idea of Yoga in specific populations.

FIVE

Gatherings: Yoga and Groups

Introduction

In this chapter we look a little closer at the premise that Yogic practices can be useful for groups of humans. When appropriate[1] forms are explored practicing yogic discipline has favorable outcomes, and although benefits are individually experienced, yogic practice can be targeted to specific groups who share conditional characteristics. The following section will delve further into the potential for yogic practices to be geared towards specific groups of individuals by looking at varieties of Yoga, the idea of Yoga for all, Yoga for all ages, Yoga for stress, and Yoga for custodial, vulnerable and post-conflict populations.

What Is Appropriate Practice?

One of the potential benefits of an exploration such as this (establishing yogic practices as a form of educating for peace) is the chance to engage with assumptions about what "doing" Yoga means. For many, "yoga" means sweating and bending in tightly fitting fitness gear for 60 to 90 minutes once or twice a week. For others, it means taking an ethical vow to practice truthfulness and nonviolence (not lying or eating meat for instance) and for others still it means using contemplative measures to attune the mind to connectivity and awareness. What can be assumed from this brief exploration is that Yoga refers to a range of practices and some clarity can be gained by briefly mentioning practices that are typical of the Yoga pantheon but not presented in the current Yogic Peace Education manual you are reading (though further editions may certainly do so): *mantra, yantra, mudras* and *kriyas*. Chapter 3 explored the classical yogic practice of *Ash-tanga* (8-limb path) as an underlying metaphysical foundation of Yogic Peace Education but in the following section we will take a quick opportunity to refer to some other practices routinely seen in the Yoga domain that could infuse Yogic Peace Educations to come: *mantra, yantra, mudras* and *kriya*.

Mantra

Sound is a transcendent vehicle for spiritual states. Mantras are sounds or vibrations that are used, similar to other yogic techniques, to focus, invite or evoke various energetic outcomes. Remember, Yoga anatomy includes a layer of *pranic* energy (the Astral Body as seen in Figure 3) that is both invisible and intimately connected to our well-being. Yogic Mantra[2] (usually but not always in Sanskrit) uses syllables uttered silently (in your mind) or audibly and repeatedly.

There are hundreds of mantras and they are used in everything from *chakra* balancing to pregnancy to inviting good fortune. The simplest mantras are called *Bija* mantras or seed sounds (see Figure 7) and each syllable is uttered to harmonize the body and energetically engage with a particular chakra.

Mantras, as was mentioned, are methods of drawing energetic focus to the *pranic* sheath by way of vibration. As the body is an energetic vessel Yoga utilizes a variety of techniques to "echo" in this vital space of wellness and mantra is beneficial to those vocalizing, mentalizing or simply listening. The passive potential of mantra means that Yoga music and devotional singing (*kirtan*), yogic chanting (audible mantra) or repetition of spoken phrases is something you can do personally or for the benefit of others within the same vibrational space. For those interested in affecting change *mantra* can present a wonderful option for transformation.

Yantra

The use of images or objects to focus the senses during meditation is a centuries-old practice. Yantras are normally images (geometric or symbolic of various deities) that are either created as a form of

Part II: Yogic Science

FIGURE 7
Bija Mantras

Chakra	Seed (*Bija*) Sound
Sahasra	Om
Ajna	Ooo
Vishuddi	Hum
Anahata	Yum
Manipura	Rum
Svadisthana	Vum
Mooladhara	Lum

concentration and single mindedness or gazed upon to induce individual states of meditation. There are some very famous yantras used in popular worship of deities but in general the benefits of yantra gazing include protection, fortitude, prosperity or salvation. A well-known ancient yantra is called the *Sri* yantra (see Figure 8).

Figure 8
***Sri* Yantra**

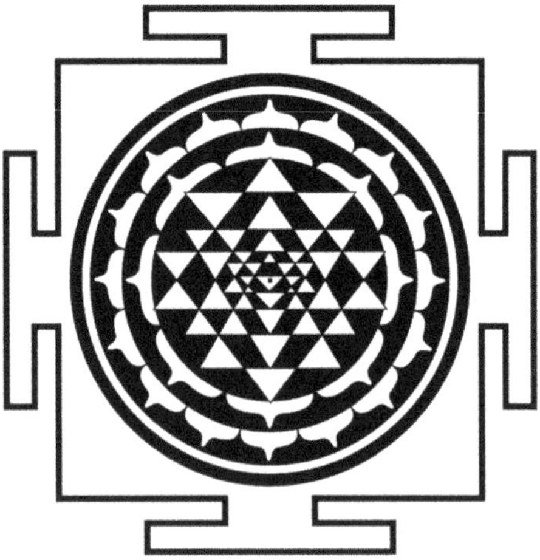

The *Sri* yantra represents the unification of the masculine and feminine in the goddess Tripura Sundari. It expresses nine levels of the universe in interlocking triangles that radiate outward from the center. Adherents who focus on the *Sri* yantra are believed to be stimulating the pituitary gland, an organ responsible for hormonal regulation.

Mudras

Mudras are sacred gestures in Yoga. In *hasta-mudra* (hand mudra) they are a simple tool for positioning hands and fingers in such a way as to invoke certain states. There are many, many mudras but some of the most common involve dexterous positions utilized in seated meditations. Common mudra include:

Dyana Mudra (Zen Mudra): hands in lap, left palm sits under right palm, tips of thumbs touching—focus is contemplation and concentration.

Anjali Mudra: hands in prayer pose (palms and fingers joined) at heart center (sternum)—focus is love and respect.

Gyana Mudra: tips of thumb and index fingers join while the remaining three fingers are lightly stretched out together—focus is concentration and knowledge

Shuni Mudra: tip of middle finger and thumb touch while other fingers relax—focus is patience and compassion.

Surya Ravi Mudra: tip of ring finger and thumb touch while other fingers relax—focus is balance and wellness.

Buddhi Mudra: tip of little finger and thumb touch while other fingers relax—focus is strength and intuition.

When people are stressed and anxious they often bunch up their hands or grip their fists together tightly. Using hand movements, gently and with breath can be a wonderful and mindful method of being present in a given moment.

Kriya

These practices can be considered "Yoga hygiene." The goal of kriya is both inner and outer cleanliness; to purify the human instrument, to maintain its efficiency and eliminate diseases of the body, mind and spirit and the space in which the body exists. Kriya can involve a collection of (possible) purification rituals that are commonly used in the practice of Yoga and include (i) nasal, dental and aural cleaning that can include use of nostril baths (*jalaneti* pots) and breathing exercises (*pranayama*), (ii) digestive cleansing that includes eating or drinking observances and restrictions and physical movements to aid in evacuation, (iii) massage and stimulation of inner organs that can involve various postures or movements, (iv) eye stimuli that include specific gazing practices, as well as (v) other physical ministrations that include modification of physical spaces, care for personal attire and belongings and hygienic practices for kriya implements. Kriya rituals are not the beginning of practice for *yogins* or simply a preparatory function of practice but an integrated and devotional commitment to Yoga as an art of optimal wellness.

These explorations of mantra, yantra, mudras and kriyas are not exhaustive but we wanted to show that there are other ways of "doing" Yoga for interested practitioners. Whole books (libraries perhaps) exist that deeply investigate the existence of known and potential mudras, yantras, mantras, etc. The goal of this short section has been to suggest that the range of yogic practices means there are ways of "doing" Yoga that many people do not entertain *off of their Yoga mats* and although there is no "one size fits all" Yoga there may be a yogic practice appropriate for everyone.

Who Benefits from Yoga?

What kind of people can benefit from Yogic Science and lifestyle practices? The short and easy answer according to Yoga teachers is that *everyone* can receive benefit with various qualifications according to the age, life stage and the health status of the person. A common decree, however, in Yoga literature relates to the frequency of practice—a person's level of dedication—and that "unless yoga is practiced regularly, sincerely and in a most disciplined manner, one does not reap the benefits" (Gore, 2005, xvii). Despite this maxim, those who dip into and out of the practice do still gain benefit, but not as great or compounding a benefit as a regular practitioner. As with many techniques or modalities of wellness, the practice of Yoga has valuable outcomes and it is common after a yogic session for practitioners to ask themselves "It feels good, I feel better, why I am not doing this more?"

Yoga was a renunciate activity in the past (where you stepped away from life and business of daily living to form a union with consciousness in a cave somewhere) but it is a lifestyle activity for many people today—an add-on if you will. As with the practice of other activities that we know are beneficial, we may have barriers that are real, imagined or due to constraints on time. For those who can afford to (in dollars and minutes) and don't have perceptible barriers to adding yogic discipline into their daily living practices, there are ample rationalizations made for why we "do not" practice: I'm busy, my back is sore, Lantheamora has a tournament, Jizanthropus isn't feeling well, I'm bloated from those nachos, I can never find a parking spot, my teacher is off sick, I forgot to wash my Yoga top, I just ate that cinnamon bun … you name it. We would do well to remove obstacles to this beneficial practice, starting with what we think Yoga "is."

Discipline, Not Dogma

In formal Yoga done with a Yoga therapist or Yoga teacher (two different Yoga professionals with two separate forms of training) a teacher will develop a suitable program for the participant in accordance with realistic goals. In this instance a dedicated professional modifies the yogic practices according to the health history, lifestyle and physiological requirements of each individual. This tailoring of the practice represents the art and science of Yoga whereby certain *asana*, *pranayama* and/or attitudinal practices are given according to the requirements of the nervous system of each person. Within classical Yoga (Raja Yoga and Hatha Yoga) one size does not fit all, yet benefit can and does frequently occur from attending group Yoga classes where individual needs do not direct the practice, but *asana*, *pranayama*, meditation and/or relaxation methods lead to increased wellbeing.

This is because Yogic Science is based upon a deep understanding of the human mind, physiology and the impact of lifestyle choices on the mind-body system. Because it is based on knowledge of one's human instrument Yogic Science is pan-cultural, pan-age and pan-gender where modifications of suitable *asana* and other yogic practices are routinely offered (Satyananda, 1966). As the body gains strength, function and flexibility daily yogic practices change which in turn alters one's daily experience of yogic practices.

And whereas Yogic Philosophy (Feuerstein, 2001) is not suitable for all cultures as it involves a metaphysical perception that is not compatible with some conceptualizations of the place of humanity in the cosmic sphere, Yogic Science, the practices, do not conflict with cultural norms or systems of thought. As a discipline based upon observations undertaken over thousands of years Yogic Science does not seek to influence the mentality of its practitioner even where certain cognitive attitudes are encouraged (such as oneness perception). As a knowledge system, Yogic Science does not claim to offer answers to injustices or inequality in human systems but offers safe techniques (Cramer et al. 2015) which can change the physiological and psychological instruments (mind and body) of practitioners, leading to gains in physical function, emotional regulation, intuition, empathy and compassion. In the following section targeted yogic discipline will be presented to include the impact of life-stages (age), dispositions (mental stress) and three special categories of individuals including individuals who are incarcerated, vulnerable individuals and post-conflict populations.

Yoga Around the Globe

We begin the process of looking at how Yoga can benefit various populations by examining how Yogic Science has been accepted around the globe. While systematic international studies are few and far between studies from the United States of America (USA), England, Australia, India and Japan contribute to understanding about how the practice is a worldwide pursuit. Cramer et al. (2016) analyzed cross-sectional data from the USA 2012 National Health Interview Survey (n=34,525) where prevalence of Yoga use and patterns of Yoga practice were analyzed. Among those who had practiced Yoga in the past 12 months, 51.2 percent attended Yoga *asana* classes, 89.9 percent used breathing exercises (*pranayama*), and 54.9 percent used meditation (*dharana or dhyana*). The reasons why people practiced Yoga included a wide variety of motivations:

78.4 percent practiced for general wellness or disease prevention,

66.1 percent practiced to improve energy,

49.7 percent practiced to improve immune function,

19.7 percent practiced to improve back pain,

6.4 percent practiced to improve stress, and,

(6.4 percent) practiced to improve arthritis (Cramer et al., 2016, 230–231).

Although Yogic Science was not specifically developed to treat disease—it was designed to promote the necessary health for optimal human spiritual and neuro-psychobiological development—many populations within Western countries have adopted Yoga techniques to manage disease and illness. Yoga Therapy, a modern modality for wellness, uses Yoga as a tool or therapy to address specific ailments and maladies in either individual practitioners or groups in need of directed healing.

According to this same study (Cramer et al., 2016) about 21 million Americans had practiced Yoga in the previous 12 months and 31 million American adults had at least some experience of Yoga. An earlier (2002) study corresponded to over 10 million adults using Yoga for health (Birdee et al., 2008) so an increase in the numbers of people utilizing Yogic Science is identified in the Cramer study doubling the popularity of the Yogic practices in the U.S. This data shows that many Americans have accepted Yoga as a modality suitable for managing health and in addition, as the specific aims of disease prevention and the relief of back pain were the most prevalent health concerns cited by participants grouped as practitioners who had only "12 months" of Yoga practice these findings can be contrasted with "lifetime" Yoga practitioners who were in better health and did not target their practice to specific ailments (Cramer et al., 2015; Birdee et al., 2008).

The use of Yoga in the U.S. shows a tendency for two kinds of practitioners: those who use Yoga for health betterment (those seen in the "12-month" group) those seen in the "lifetime" group characterized by the following traits: female, younger, non–Hispanic white, college educated, higher earners, living in the West, and of better health (Cramer et al., 2015, 230–231; Birdee et al., 2008).

As we can see, while Yogic Science was developed for all human beings these studies suggest that there are certain groups in the U.S.

who are "using" Yoga to treat health issues and certain groups who are more open to routinizing yogic practice and therefore experiencing better health. A similar demographic picture has been shown in England. Ding and Stamatakis (2014) analyzed the prevalence of Yoga in England by taking the 2013 Health Survey for England data and examining independent adult cohorts for the years 1997–1999; 2003–2004; and 2006–2008. They uncovered that those practicing Yoga were likely to be older, female, University degree educated, non-manual labor workers, with low Body Mass Index, better self-rated general health, inactive employment, and with a lifestyle including higher moderate to vigorous physical activity. The prevalence of Yoga (measured as a practice undertaken in the previous four weeks) was determined for each cohort studies showing a significant increase in the Yoga use and popularity (0.46 percent 1997–1998; 0.94 percent 2003–2004; 1.11 percent 2006–2008).

A hemisphere away in Australia a very similar demographic picture is suggested. Penman et al. (2012) conducted a national online survey of 2,567 self-selected Yoga practitioners and found that the typical respondent was aged 41, tertiary educated, employed (full-time, part-time or self-employed), health conscious and female. Most respondents practiced *vinyasa* Yoga followed by relaxation, breathing (*pranayama*), or meditation (*dharana, dhyana*). Males were more likely to practice vigorous "physical Yoga" such as various forms of hot Yoga. In this study of self-selected *yogins* (Yoga practitioners) over half of the group practiced once or twice a week (56.6 percent), while 24.1 percent practiced three to four sessions per week.

India is the birthplace of Yogic Science and in 2011 Nayak et al. surveyed the use of stress reduction techniques of 904 adults, over twenty years of age, in the city of Ahmedabad, Gujarat, India. In this study roughly ⅓ of the surveyed group was practicing what was described as "stress reduction techniques" (34.3 percent) and 90 percent of the "stress reduction group" practiced daily. The stress reduction practices included:

(i) Religious practices (mantra, chanting, *dhyana*, prayer, spiritual book reading, rituals and listening to music) (78.4 percent)
(ii) *Asana* Yoga (11.6 percent)
(iii) Meditation (4.8 percent).

Those practicing stress reduction techniques were more likely to be females over the age of forty, college educated, in a sedentary occupation, from upper and middle class backgrounds, married, and less likely to have diabetes and hypertension (as compared with those who do not practice stress reduction). This profile of the demographic population practicing Yoga for stress reduction in India gives a similar picture to the available data from the U.S., England and Australia identifying the most prevalent type of Yoga practitioner as female. Also, the sort of activities used in stress reduction differed internationally; techniques of physical postures (*asana*), breathing (*pranayama*) and meditation (*dharana, dhyana*) predominated Yogic practice in the U.S. study, while the majority of practitioners in the Indian sample used non-physical practices.

A Japanese study in 2015 by Miyata et al. testing mindfulness and the psychological status of Yoga practitioners referenced two Japanese-language studies that state the estimated number of Japanese Yoga practitioners increased threefold from 2006 to 2010 from 330,000 to 1,000,000 (Ito, 2011; Nagashima, 2012). While the lack of English translation of their work makes it difficult for researchers who do not understand Japanese to understand the root of such statistics, it nonetheless suggests an increase in Yoga practice similar to other global centers. As Yoga becomes more prevalent internationally more studies are needed to locate how and in what way Yogic Science is utilized but from the limited data located in this exploration it seems that Yoga is predominantly a gendered activity for those middle aged with good education and income.

This perhaps reflects the fact that in several countries Hatha Yoga is not currently part of an integrated Yogic lifestyle, but rather is mostly experienced as a series of group classes entailing free time and some level of disposable income. Ashrams in India offering Hatha Yoga training involve expensive tuition; costly airfares and four-week training periods that may represent the entirety of annual leave for most gainfully employed adults. Such integrated Yoga experiences can be financially prohibitive, geographically remote and temporally unavailable to many would-be *yogins*. Holistic (Raja Yoga) techniques are usually community and ashram-based whereas in the West such yogic infrastructure is undeveloped or nonexistent to community practitioners. For this reason, Raja Yoga is less well studied and utilized in Western

Yoga. To reflect this disposition, most modern studies have not sought to view Yoga as an integrated science but a collection of techniques found independently (like a buffet) but disconnected from classical Yoga foundations.

Yoga: Best for Whom?

As we consider whom Yogic Science might benefit, it is useful to reiterate that Yoga is a term covering a range of practices; Hatha Yoga is the combination of *asana* (physical postures) and *pranayama* (breathing techniques) whereas Raja Yoga includes the previous practices but adds techniques that include ethical tenets (*yama/niyama*), mental focus (*dharana*) and meditation (*dhyana*) techniques.

Now that we are versed in the breadth of the most common forms of Yogic Science we might assume that yogic exercises are beneficial for all those who chose to practice them. But what about adverse side effects of Yogic practice? Of unfavorable and unexpected—not to mention unwanted—experiences that may have resulted from yogic practices? A growing body of evidence suggests that although *asana* are predominantly safe physical injuries were identified in a Japanese survey that gives some clearer information regarding Yoga as potentially detrimental. In a 2015 study Matsushita and Oka surveyed 2508 people (and 271 Yoga therapists) who were asked about adverse events that occurred during Yoga class where "adverse" events were generally defined as unwelcome symptoms that happened during practice in a Yoga class experienced *on the same day* the survey was distributed. Of those attending a Yoga class, 53.5 percent had chronic diseases and 42.3 percent were receiving medication from hospitals. Of this same group 27.8 percent reported the experience of an adverse symptom during class; that most events were mild (63.8 percent), that the symptom did not stop further participation or comprised and obstacle to completing the class. Of the reported "adverse" symptoms the most common were myalgia (muscle pain) and/or musculoskeletal symptoms such as aching, stiffness or fatigue.

What this study showed was that risk factors for adverse events were significantly higher for practitioners suffering from chronic disease, poor physical condition (on the day), and in those who felt that the class was either physically or mentally stressful. Events that interfered with ongoing Yoga practice were common in the elderly (70<) and those with chronic musculoskeletal diseases. This suggests that Yoga classes for those who are elderly or who are experiencing chronic disease in Japan may require modification.

In another recent Japanese study (Miyata et al. 2015) the psychological and mindfulness effects of integrated Hatha Yoga (poses and breathing techniques) were investigated against Raja Yoga techniques (focused attention-based meditation) in populations who routinely practiced classical Yogic Science (from 0.3 to 34.0 years). Miyata et al. reported that,

> Compared with age and sex-matched control participants, yoga practitioners self-reported significantly higher scores on mindfulness, well-being, positive affect, and empathy, and lower scores on depression and negative affect. Among the practitioners ... the amount of yoga/meditation practice, regardless of ages, predicted higher scores on mindfulness and well-being and lower scores on depression, negative affect, and empathy [2015, 560].

This study as it shows that the *frequency* and *duration* of Yoga is significantly implicated in increases in wellbeing and positive psychological change.

In contrast to Japan, in India it is unlikely that such people would be invited to attend group Yoga classes. Instead, persons suffering from chronic illness or age related symptoms would consult a Yoga therapist skilled in assessing wellness, modifying *asana* and prescribing a suitable set of *vinyasa* based on individual need. In India, it is the responsibility of a Yoga therapist to ensure that the yogic practices prescribed are safe and suitable for the individual seeking help.

In Yoga Therapy a specialist offers a careful observational assessment including but not limited to: joint movement (ease, range, direction, compensation, skin temperature over the joint, tenderness over the joint, muscle bulk, tone, strength and smoothness of movement, palpitation of upper back, signs of lordosis (inward spinal curvature) and kyphosis (outward spinal curvature) (Chandrasekaran, 2012). Such situations then lead to recommendations concerning specific physical conditions and symptoms for example the instruction not to, "practice any inverted asanas if there is gas or fermentation in the intestines, if the blood is excessively impure, during menstruation or in later stages of pregnancy" (Satyananda, 1966, 17). As many the regretful *yogin* understands (remembering that breakfast burrito you had just before class once) *asana* practices were originally designed to occur on an empty stomach and at the beginning of the day. The reasons concerned the aforementioned gastrointestinal dilemma of asking the body to focus on digestion during yogic exercises, and that certain *asana* are not suitable to be practiced in the evening as they may affect the sleep cycle.

This accords with statements of classical Indian Yoga teachers that if, "yoga is practiced regularly, sincerely and in a most disciplined manner," one can reap many benefits (Gore, 2005, xvii). If regular practice creates health and personality changes claimed in the ancient yogic texts and empirically witnessed in various global locales, then perhaps yogic discipline can be a beneficial practice for particular subpopulations of interest. The "one size does not fit all but it may be beneficial for many" conversation continues with the next section that looks closer at the appropriateness of yogic discipline at various developmental stages of the life cycle.

Yoga for All?

Traditionally, India Yogic Science was considered useful for all ages because it formed a breadth of exercises and techniques that were harmless and helpful. In "well" populations Yoga involves a complete system of practice but, according to age and health, yogic discipline may involve Yoga Therapy with a program that is modified for individual circumstances. In the West there is the common perception that Yoga practices are increasing in popularity and that a large segment of Western populations are now adding yogic discipline to their lifestyle choices. We cannot currently "know" (from the limited empirical investigations that stand) if the practice of Yogic Science is pervasive but studies do show that Yoga is proving popular amongst a small population sub-set, namely older, well educated, women and this demographic reality is echoed in a number of studies as mentioned in the previous section (Cramer et al., 2016; Birdee et al., 2008; Ding and Stamatakis, 2014). What we also know is that by 2007, upward of 1.5 million children were participating in Yoga programs across the United

States and if one Googles "Yoga for kids" one can reasonably assume this figure is increasing with "search results" of over 118,000,000 hits (Barnes, Bloom, and Nahin, 2009).

But an increase in the prevalence and practice of Yoga in the west is not always rooted in the Science of Yoga as understood in classical training. In India, yogic exercises are only considered suitable for children from mid-childhood onward.

Surya namaskar (translated as "salute to the sun') is a physical series (a *vinyasa*) of twelve flowing postures including alternating forward and backward movements. This *vinyasa* is said to stretch the spinal column and massage vital organs by alternately bending the body forwards and backwards. The *vinyasa* of *surya namaskar* uses mindful breathing—of inhalation (*puracka*) and exhalation (*rechaka*)—that increases oxygenation in our lungs, which then act to distribute vital energy to the cells of the body. The rhythm of breathing (inhaling as the body opens and exhaling as the body closes) becomes natural and rhythmic which further increases the benefits of chemical exchange (oxygen-carbon dioxide) in the cellular structures of our physique detoxifying the body and invigorating the whole human instrument. Our bodies have three methods whereby toxins and pollutants are removed from the body: perspiration, evacuation and *expiration*. Because *surya namaskar* involves a dedicated practice of inhalation and exhalation it has a deep effect in detoxifying the body by oxygenating our cells (once you fully breathe out you can then more abundantly breathe in oxygenated air) with the added benefit of regulating emotions and providing practitioners with a deep feeling of relaxation (Singh et al., 2010).

The classical Yoga teacher is encouraged to make Yoga training fun and enjoyable for the young. In addition to the age and physical development of a juvenile student particular awareness is focused on a child's stage of spiritual progress, constructing equilibrium between introspection and gregariousness.

Indeed, this awareness of such inner psychology relates to a recent study by Weaver and Darragh (2015) who found that Yoga training was very useful for children and adolescents experiencing anxiety. The authors conducted a systematic review of anxiety reduction in children and adolescents indicating less anxiety from those practicing Yoga. The variable outcome measures and study populations limit the generalizability of this review but nevertheless, show positive benefits for young practitioners from yogic practices (Weaver and Darragh, 2015).

In addition to suitability for the young Indian teachers see yogic discipline as safe and advantageous for the elderly. Gururaja et al. (2011) investigated the effects of Yoga in comparative age cohorts. A small number of people (n=25) were placed into groups according to age; fifteen people aged between 65 to 75 years and 10 people aged between 20 to 30 years. They all participated in 90 minutes of Yoga classes once or twice a week for one month. Both groups had significant reductions in both state and trait anxiety.

Kim et al. (2015) compared the effect of combined pelvic muscle and yogic exercises on urinary incontinence in middle aged women, recruited from a community health center in Seoul, Korea. Over eight weeks, thirty-four women completed the twice-weekly Yoga program and results showed significant improvements in attitude toward pelvic muscle exercises, pelvic muscle strength, and incontinence factors. Daily performance of pelvic muscle exercise was positively correlated with improved incontinence factors and "quality of life" related to urinary tract symptoms.

Like many of the studies identified in this chapter further scientific enquiry is needed, controlling specifically for chance and the mixing of techniques but despite these flaws we can see that the wellness fields are beginning to examine the usefulness of Yoga according to age and age-related health complaints. In general, findings would be assisted by greater methodological consistency and much larger sample sizes but as a lay reader it is safe to conclude that Yoga can be helpful ideally in conjunction with the Indian recommendation of working with a trained Yoga teacher or therapist.

Classical Yoga maintains that Yoga is useful for "all" because despite the fixation on fitness and ability (and agility) in the West, yogic discipline is not merely *asana* practice (physical postures) and Yogic Science makes no requirements that practitioners have particular abilities of any sort. Indeed one could practice *mantra*, *mudra*, mental training (*dharana*, *dhyana*), breath control (*pranayama*) or ethical restraints and observances (*yamas* or *niyamas*) and still be "doing" perfectly suitable (and overwhelmingly beneficial) Yoga. The reliance on varieties (modifications) of "hundreds" of poses is also counter to many schools of Yoga that only really use some few poses daily, over long periods of time.

> [Yoga] books list eighty-four postures (āsanas) altogether, but many of them are rarely used, some perhaps never. There are about a dozen of the gymnastic ones which are frequently used and which, in fact, would more than cover the ground required for health and functioning (in contrast with the partial atrophy so common in modern life) of all parts of the body [Wood, 159, 114].

So, despite the emphasis on the physical practices of Yoga, many poses are rarely, if ever, utilized (much less taught), and only a small number (about a dozen) comprise the basic postures typical in Hatha Yoga *asana* practice. Yogic Science is a complete system of living with a wide variety of "types" of Yoga (based on the suitability of each to each and every practitioners) and practice options to enhance well-being. And so, depending upon your human instrument (body-mind-spirit) practicing Yoga could mean a wide variety of exercises and mindsets used where appropriate over the arch of the whole lifecycle. While certain traditions of physical sequences are not suitable for all (populations experiencing everything from pregnancy, chronic disability, mental distress to injury, illness or other common maladies) there is always an available form of Yoga to "do." Classical Yoga would introduce specific practices where appropriate and under suitable and capable supervision and instruction. The answer to "Is Yoga for all?" is yes, but not all forms of Yoga, and not all the time.

Yoga for Stress

All yogic practices are designed to ease the effects of tension and stress which is good as scientists suggest that most human beings living in modern cities (and in the 21st century we are living increasingly in urban centers as a species) are both physiologically and psychologically stressed. At an intuitive level we agree with this assertion. As we find ourselves sitting in traffic, cued up at a bureaucracy, sitting in a classroom, perhaps at an office desk or other work environment we can forget that the physical body is often suffering. Sometimes we lose awareness of the tightness in our muscles, an angle in our necks, the feeling of our feet, the effects of prolonged concentration on the brain, or the constant worry of being a human in inhuman spaces. We may forget that our bodies and nervous systems did not evolve in environments that required lots of sitting. It can be easy to forget that the early lifestyle for human beings did not involve furniture; "In the natural, simple life people would normally sit on grass or earth, not on hard rocks or boards. The natural cushioning flesh on the human buttocks indicates the need for some softness, but does not sufficiently provide against hard material" (Wood, 1958, 113). Many of us find ourselves sitting on furniture that is too small, too soft, too hard or too big for our frames. We can find ourselves spending hours in traffic jammed in vehicles that are not made to fit our physical forms. One size does not fit all, yet in the modern post-industrial world we pretend that it does. Indeed we have forgotten that it used to be any different.

The basis of Yoga is to create a base of calm and relaxation within the human being to strengthen our ability to release acquired tension and emotionally regulate our feelings through conscious awareness.

> Relaxation plays a great part in yoga technique. In the shavāsana one can perhaps learn it as completely as possible. But the general idea is that when one part of the body is being used, the other parts should be as relaxed as much as may be practicable. One form of relaxation is often neglected, that of the face, which should certainly be performed along with general relaxation before going to sleep [Wood, 1959, 116].

How many times a day do we make time to rest, to relax, to let go of everything that came before a moment of repose? The reality is that we should be making time each day (many times a day ideally) to rest and relax and find an outlet for our tensions and stress. Imagine a world where checking your emails was less important than affecting a posture of repose for five minutes every hour. The truth is, we cannot expect the "cup of tension" not to overflow if we do not regularly empty it. If stress was a rain barrel and it rained for days, months (years?) at a time you know it would overflow. Stress is an overflowing rain barrel. Yoga is a release of tension; it is designed to regularly empty the space we hold stress. We all experience stress, and different levels of stress, differently. We have multiple terms for stress in our world and often categorize ourselves by our degree of stress. We suffer from anxiety, nervousness, apprehension, concern, worry, fear, unease, angst, fretfulness, uncertainly, trepidation, foreboding, distress, dread, agony, anguish, dismay, terror –the list goes on, and on, and on like words for snow in the Inuit language. The "we" of Yoga for stress is the "we" of humanity. The stress-free human probably does exist, maybe because they got the last parking spot, the last donut, the last spot on the ferry boat, they made it to work on time, to their child's soccer game, paid all the bills this month or some other temporary, momentary, release from the relentless. The rest of us, we need Yoga. And some of us *really* need Yoga. The following sections will briefly touch on three important human groups we consider in our exploration of gatherings and Yogic Peace Education: incarcerated, vulnerable and post-conflict populations.

Custodial Practice: Yoga for Incarcerated Populations

As Yoga becomes more popular in the West we have seen it move into the arena of *management* and perhaps *rehabilitation* for people incarcerated in prison systems. While well-designed social science studies are few and far between, there are some interesting findings. Bilderbeck et al., 2013, designed a randomized controlled trial of Yoga across seven British prisons where over ten weeks inmates attended once-weekly Hatha Yoga sessions that lasted two hours. Both before and after the ten-week program participants were assessed in areas including perceived stress, executive control, positive and negative effects, and psychological distress. Compared to a control group (who did not practice Yoga) the Yoga participants manifested decreased levels of both perceived stress and psychological distress.

This finding is not surprising given the general claims and research supporting Yoga as a calming practice. What is of interest to Yogic Peace Education is that the Yoga group showed higher levels of positivity and executive control after the 10-week intervention. So, not only did those in the Yoga group experience less stress personally, they became physiologically calmer and psychologically positive—in a highly stressful prison environment this is a very beneficial outcome for incarcerated individuals and those who work with them.

Less stress, more positive, but what does "executive control" mean? According to Hillman et al., "executive control refers to a subset of cognitive processes involved in the intentional component of environmental interaction and includes functions relating to the organization of action, mental flexibility, complex discrimination, error monitoring, response selection, and inhibition" (2004, 176). This is not a "feeling" of wellbeing, or the disposition of being "chilled out"; this is a shift in cognitive functioning. This does not necessarily mean that violent people become less violent, but that after only two hours of Yoga a week they have more *choice* over their actions—they are more aware and less reactive in their environments (a gain all Yoga students obtain).

Studies confirm that cardiovascular exercise and physical activity benefit executive function in adults (Colcombe and Kramer, 2003). But, when Yoga *asanas* are practiced breathing and metabolism *slows down* whereas during physical exercise "breath and metabolism speed up, oxygen consumption rises, and the body gets hot ... [so while] yoga postures tend to arrest the catabolism (break down of cells) ... exercise promotes it," so whereas activity in general is good and has a positive outcome on executive function (not to mention our other physiological and psychological systems) Yoga is an activity option that provides all of the advantages of physical exercise without the disadvantages of catabolism (Satyananda, 1966, 12).

More than the physical benefits of yogic practices classical Yoga *asanas* were a way to obtain an integrated nervous system capable of the practices of meditation. There is a growing literature in the West that supports the claim that yogic practices changes our brains and that the brain and its neural systems are capable of modification in response to various forms of physical and mental training (Hölzel et al., 2011; Luders et al., 2011; Luders et al., 2012; Lutz et al., 2009). In meditation we begin to see increases in the structure of the hippocampal region responsible for memory and emotional regulation (Luders et al., 2009) and people begin to develop the neural pathways necessary for empathy, psychological wellbeing and compassion (Singleton et al., 2014). In people suffering from depression and post-traumatic stress disorder (PTSD), brain imaging has shown less grey matter in the hippocampal region and more grey matter in the medulla region—the part of the brain responsible for flight-fight-freeze and threat and self-protection reflexes. One study on Hatha Yoga, (*pranayama* and *asana*), found that Yoga could effectively treat symptoms of (PTSD) (van der Kolk, 2006) that can include flashbacks, nightmares or feelings of depression and anxiety.

Another interesting study examined the re-incarceration rates of 190 imprisoned persons who had completed an Ananda Marga Yoga course while in custody (Landau and Gross, 2008). In this study jailed individuals were separated into two groups according to how many Yoga sessions they had attended (4+ or 1–3). The Yoga group (n=52) was the term used to describe those who had attended four or more classes and the non–Yoga group (n=138) included those who had attended only one to three classes. Following a median post-release period of 18 months (with a range of 1 to 58 months), only 8.5 percent of the Yoga group was re-incarcerated, compared to 25.2 percent in the non–Yoga group (over a median of 12 months, post-release range of 6 to 31 months). Findings such as these indicate that the connection between Yoga programs and these kinds of situational changes for incarcerated peoples are important and possibly very fruitful areas for further inquiry.

Yoga and Vulnerable Populations

The American Journal of Managed Care (AJMC) considers a vulnerable population to include:

> The economically disadvantaged, racial and ethnic minorities, the uninsured, low-income children, the elderly, the homeless, those with human immunodeficiency virus (HIV), and those with other chronic health conditions, including severe mental illness. It may also include rural residents, who often encounter barriers to accessing healthcare services. The vulnerability of these individuals is enhanced by race, ethnicity, age, sex, and factors such as income, insurance coverage (or lack thereof), and absence of a usual source of care. Their health and healthcare problems intersect with social factors, including housing, poverty, and inadequate education [AJMC, 2006, 1].

Vulnerable populations include all ages, all genders, all races and all ethnicities and ability levels. The goal of this short section is not to lump all of these very diverse individuals into meta-groups (for example, all women or all children or all persons living with a mental illness) but to suggest that there may be a therapeutic role for yogic practices for individuals who suffer from various hindrances.

One recent study by Ikai et al. (2013) designed an eight-week single-blind randomized controlled analysis examining the effects of Yoga training on postural stability in outpatients with schizophrenia or related psychotic disorders (ICD-10). This is a recent study that connects the practice of Yoga to persons considered vulnerable and the findings are very hopeful. In Ikai et al.'s results, they showed significant improvements in the Yoga group on length of trunk motion (flexibility, strength and speed of the body trunk), the Romberg ratio (ability to balance with eyes closed), and anteflexion (the ability to bend forward) at week eight. This study looked at physiological improvement using Yoga but other investigations could look at standard practices (not the all-encompassing term Yoga) such as asana or pranayama exercise. In such studies there may be a rich area for future enquiry into the efficacy of Yogic Peace Education, as practices presented in this manual could be used in a baseline study for further investigations into Yoga in vulnerable populations.

Yoga Post-Conflict

Peace and Conflict Studies (a discipline that includes peace education) is committed to identifying violence in society and transforming conflict without violence. In this field there is an ongoing conversation of the values of programs that are international interventions that embody the tenets of Galtung's concept of Negative Peace (cessation of direct violence), humanitarian pursuits that address hunger, disease, housing and basic needs and developmental initiatives that seek to support livelihoods and governance infrastructures. It is not "instead of" any of these interventions that Yogic Peace Education would be best utilized but rather in addition to other programs that seek to address physical wellbeing, mental health (trauma healing for example), traditional or indigenous peacebuilding (reconciliation and mediation) or strategies of inter-communal peacebuilding (where previously conflictual parties bridge divides to find shared humanity). In communities where groups of individuals have experienced trauma (as either victims or perpetrators or both) there should be space for transformative exercises such as those described in Yogic Peace Education. The authors, in coalescing this information into a theory and practice manual, look forward to frontline peacebuilders (in any contexts) sharing their discoveries with us in the future.

Five. Gatherings

KATERINA: I want to mention something that really echoes in my mind: those (often able-bodied and resource-rich) with the privilege of making positive life choices do so from a place of possibility that is often denied to others. This relates to growing, buying and consuming food, making time to attend holistically to personal wellbeing and the wellbeing of others and the "culture clash," "time crunch" or "technology tethers" that take away (or seem to) one's feeling of positively administering to the needs of one's, body, mind and spirit.

Sometimes (but not always) those who would benefit most from Yogic Science (and myriad other wellness modalities and resources) are unable to do so because the cost (in either minutes or dollars) of the practice is prohibitive. But that compartmentalization of Yoga is missing a great big opportunity to viralize Yoga (if you will forgive the epidemiological metaphor) so that Yoga is not a "thing" each individual does (or sells or buys) on their own but something that is spread by people within and between groups and collectives "for each other," not simply to benefit the self. Yoga means, union: joining or yoking together (people, cells, and consciousness) so the mindset of practice is critical. Yoga "with" is Yoga. Yoga "for" is Yoga too. Even if my Yoga is personal, private and uncommunicated I am merging my energy with the energy of the whole world so I am both together and apart. As they say in maya-vada Yoga, "my separate-ness from you is an illusion." But my thinking on this is an "idea" and I understand that many other people don't share this idea. The compartmentalization keeps us all going to the grocery store to buy food we should be growing ourselves. But those that don't know how to garden (me for instance) and those who don't know how to breathe need support, we need education, we need education(s) that make us more human, not less.

JANINE: Yes. And somewhere these ideas became denigrated as hippie, somehow marketed in the eighties as quaint and irrelevant. I have never really understood that. I was even shocked when my kids would say "mum you're such a hippie." I mean, how did that happen? I have been an accountable member of society for years. So when did my ideas become so radical? I realize that they were simply the values that I grew up with a short forty years ago. That it was right to grow your own food. We didn't question it. That making our own clothes and appreciating the provision of nature was a smart way to live. That food did not come out of the garden looking the same shape, size or color; even from the same plant. We accepted that along with the need to wash the dirt off. We watched our parents compost food scraps and look after the soil so that the quality of vegetables and fruit stayed nice. I watched my parents collect seed and gather fruit from wild roadside trees. Certain times of the year were great because that was when certain fruits were available—in their correct season with no forcing of production; no year round availability. We grew up aware of nature because we were closer and more reliant on her. Sometimes we were uncomfortable yet hardly ever over full in our stomachs. In some ways this is another form of yama/niyama—just simple life style habits. We were taught to walk places rather than take the car. It meant that we developed awareness because we had to do things more slowly and live more locally.

Conclusions

This brief section looked at the notion of practicing Yoga for, by and with other people. The truth is, one size does not fit all, and despite the popularity of the eight-limb path devised by Patanjali and enshrined in the *Yoga Sutras*, yogic practices contain a great many methodologies and techniques. Regardless of the modality employed by different groups, what these forms share is the outcomes of yogic practices: physiological, psychological and energetic beneficial transformation. The previous section looked further into the potential for yogic practices to be geared towards specific groups of individuals because, as was mentioned, although there is no "one size fits all" Yoga there may be a yogic practice for everyone. The deep effects of Yoga lead to balance within each human being and will be discussed more fully in the next chapter.

SIX

Learning Peace

Introduction

"Those who hope to work for peace in the world must themselves be striving for a sense of inner harmony" (Harris and Morrison, 2013, 15). The following content seeks to give learners tangible skills (separated into three toolkits) to holistically harmonize the self. The goal of the following section is not to simply "activate" the potential of Yogic Peace Education but to encourage learners to look inward in advance of outward actions.

The science of yogic wellness involves an appreciation of the energetic nature of the universe. There are things we cannot see that have enormous impact on the quality of our lives and the quality of our interactions with one another. If we consider that life is the result of energy acting on matter—or a divine spark—we can easily recognize that there is a life force or power potential that contributes to the vital potency that animates us. *Prana* (as indicated in Chapter Three) is life force—the lightest manifestation of matter and the heaviest expression of the spirit[1]—and the accumulation of *prana* increases our wellness; wellness is something we tangibly experience in our bodies, our relationships and our communities. Yogic Peace Education involves recognizing, generating, conserving and securing *prana*. Yet it is not a process of seeking to have more *prana* (as in: *more power*), it is rather the process of embodying a peaceful apparatus for vitality that naturally permits the accumulation of the life force (*prana*) in myriad ways.

We are the peaceful apparatus or regulated neuro-psychobiological system that *prana* expresses itself through. *We* become the embodiment or presence of non-animosity, life nourishment or *ahimsa*. In a balanced state *we* naturally have more energy or *prana*. In this chapter we identify the knowledge convergence between peace education and Yogic Science and we outline the Yogic processes of attaining *prana* using the Yogic Peace Education Learning, Living and Loving Toolkits.

Yogic Peace Education is Yogic Peacebuilding

Peacebuilding is an intervention that creates nonviolent, life nourishing change. It seems that the qualities that are necessary for a peacebuilder are well known but what is less clear is how to enable the student to embody these qualities in the face of day-to-day life pressures. From a yogic perspective the practices leading to natural nonviolence and life nourishment are codified and well documented. For peacebuilders, simply adding Yogic Peace Education to their capabilities and understanding becomes an opportunity to express nonviolent practices in all facets of daily living. Similar to moving slowly when waking from slumber, there are various ways a person can gently enter the practices of Yogic Peace Education on the way to being an instrument of wellness. The following section will introduce the five principles of yogic peace education, ways of entering the practice of Yogic peace education, and then develop the capacities of Yogic Peace Education through the learning, living, and loving toolkits.

Five Principles of Yogic Peace Education

A natural agreement exists about what qualities are considered important in the development of peacebuilders in peace education and Yogic Science. The elements that comprise the convergences between both disciplines become the five guiding principles in Yogic Peace Education; each relates to various observances and restraints from the peace paradigm that relate to practice (see Table 4).

Practice refers to actions, words or mindsets that are consciously and mindfully exercised instead of reactionary or thoughtless actions. Such repetition creates peace habits that are readily available and con-

TABLE 4
Peacebuilding Values in Yoga and Peace Education

Peace Education	Yogic Science
1. Integrity: Unity, authenticity, neither lying nor taking what belongs to others	1. *Satya* 2. *Asteya*
2. Nonviolence Compassion for all things, refraining from harming others, resisting self-destructive behavior	3. *Ahimsa*
3. Simplicity: Sustainability, moderation, clean-living, contentment, letting go of things, self-control	4. *Bramacharya* 5. *Saucha* 6. *Aparigraha*
4. Connection: To spirit, God or universal consciousness, Practicing the art of contentment and appreciating the "bigger" picture (the "omnipresent" not just the "I")	7. *Santosha* 8. *Isvarapranidhara*
5. Consciousness: Self-Awareness, working to reveal the truth with vigor and compassion	9. *Tapas* 10. *Svadyaya*

tribute to compassionate living. When we encounter life (thoughts, experiences or materials) we can use the Yogic Peace Education toolkits to make dynamic and healthful choices. When we utilize Yogic Peace Education we choose the peace option, the nonviolent route and the pathway to *prana*.

Tips for Teachers, Facilitators and Yogic Peacebuilders

We are teacher/facilitators, both of us, with decades of planning, marking, delivery and aspirations between us. On top of that we have taught in educational and recreational settings where willing and less willing recipients have come to share in our offerings. We intimately understand that some students come to us by choice and some by circumstance and no two students are the same (whether in culture, learning, personality or disposition).

Further, those of us who facilitate and/or teach face significant obstacles to create, fill, maintain and foster learning environments that support "it" (whatever "it" is) to happen. There are numerous complications to teaching and lots of obstacles to teaching *peace* but for those who seek to become yogic peacebuilders (or add Yogic Peace Education to their teaching toolkits) some mention must be made of the problems teachers face when introducing yogic science to communities and individuals who hold disparate metaphysical views and dissimilar ideological sensibilities. Skeptics are difficult, believers are challenging and in either situation your best defense against resistance to introducing these exercises is *your own practice.* You cannot share the water if you, yourself are not comfortable going to the well so in all seriousness, if you want to share Yogic Peace Education then practice it yourself: *embody the content you intend to share.*

For those engaging with a prejudice against yogic science and Yogic Peace Education because of a perception that it is either a cult or religion and/or damaging or dangerous to established faith systems the following communications may be useful (please modify as needed).

LONG LETTER TO PARENT OR GUARDIAN

Dear Parent (or guardian),

Your (son or daughter) has expressed interest in participating in a unit of learning called Yogic Peace Education. Yogic Peace Education uses specific learning tools to increase the ability of your (son or daughter) to encounter difficulty and/or conflict from a place of resilience, strength and grace. The goal of this unit is to increase your child's capacity to self-regulate stress, limit feelings of detachment and depression and increase their natural, healthy ability to balance mental and emotional fluctuations. Participation is voluntary and your child is welcome to ask questions, join in or opt out of any or all of the exercises. This unit involves practical techniques including breathing and mental calming, is non-harming, has no cost, requires no preparation and needs no additional materials. Questions are welcome.

SHORT LETTER TO PARENT OR GUARDIAN

Our class is engaging in Yogic Peace Education this term. This includes learning methods that contribute to personal well-being and intellectual capabilities. These techniques will involve mindfulness (contemplation and/or meditation) and neurophysiological exercises (breathing and/or movement) expressly designed to help students manage stress and maximize their learning potential. Questions are welcome.

Six. Learning Peace

There are many learning units that challenge us as teachers and students, and although you can seek to do no harm in sharing information, you cannot know the full extent of impact of anything you do. In clarity and straightforward communication, you can simply engage with others, build relationships (to people and ideas) and start the conversation. We encourage teacher and facilitators to work from a place of nonviolent love and kindness in all endeavors and to practice caring of self and others. There are good ideas for doing something and equally good ideas for *not* doing so. Listen to your instincts, work from a place of wellness (that means practice) and gather wisdom as it comes. And remember, it is only ever the first time once—you are learning too.

JANINE: I seldom introduce yogic techniques as "Yoga" although I do honor and acknowledge the traditions and cultures that yogic ideas come from. What I have learned is to make it practical and linked to narratives that students can relate to. For example; I remember working in the field in Asia with a dedicated team of local young people. I noticed that the young people working to better their communities were also simultaneously struggling with painful stiff bodies. Many were struggling with breathing difficulties and wheezing due to heat and pollution. The journeys into the villages were a long distance, by very rough roads in extremely high temperatures. This kind of living and travel hurts the body. One night in the dark during an electricity outage I taught them how to relax their bodies, calm their minds and reduce the pain. We looked at simple breathing techniques that reduced the wheeze in their bodies and certain breathing techniques from Yoga that are known to cool the body. It was fun and practical and necessary. This kind of narrative is useful for those who are planning to work directly in community peacebuilding. It then makes sense for the student to practice gaining these skills and abilities because the tools are readily demonstrable without "belief" or "faith" in something. When a person breaths into only the left nostril—the body cools, the evidence is immediate, personal, observable and unfiltered by outside perception. There is no sleight of hand or trickery and it is relevant to the moment so it is appropriate.

Within University and formal classroom settings I seek agreement. At the beginning of each semester we form an accord in terms of how we (in the class) wish to communicate with each other and what non-conflictual communication skills we will practice (regardless of the academic topic). I explain that I will integrate practical ideas and skills for managing our personal levels of stress resulting from doing community work. In academic fora I understand that some of us are learning about international conflict and/or politics in order to make some positive difference in the world. I then state that the base of any outside change is our own inner state of composure and personal neural wiring. We then begin class with a simple "sitting in silence," tuning in our minds. We end the class in a similar way.

If it is an actual Yoga workshop in a peacebuilding class, then we end by talking about field work and the importance of keeping a strong body in difficult environments. For students with a strong faith and religious practice many of these ideas will be held within their traditions, for example: importance of prayer, silence, contemplation and willingness to serve and work towards justice. For students without a religious base then their experience of techniques can be understood in neuro-physiological manner. With either type of student, the techniques are non-harming, beneficial and easy to incorporate into routines.

KATERINA: My students in college and university settings often resist new pedagogy and learning outcomes because they are uncertain how to achieve excellent outputs (we know that students are motivated by marks and often ignore other types of outcomes). And, some of my students have refused to participate in "arrival" or "tuning in" exercises when I introduce them because contemplative techniques can be new or different and many students are wary and uncertain, which makes them apprehensive and anxious. In my experience, there are always those ready to try something new (jump right in) and those that need to watch other people swim before they get in the water. This is just fine. I think it is important to give space to all kinds of people and make participation in yogic peace education practice invitational and optional. I ask students to either close their eyes or look down, and if they would rather not join in with my cues and suggestions they are free to grocery shop in their minds or mentally redecorate their fantasy chalet if they so choose. I try to put my students at ease because they are very concerned with failing at something they are unfamiliar with and I have no desire to add to their list of "I can't" in any way.

I will often ask students to entertain the fact that they are 100 percent proficient in a capability they probably take for granted: breathing. If they are alive in my classroom they have successfully breathed (to the point of survival) their ENTIRE lives, they are already good at breathing, and I am just going to offer some tips for using something they are already good at to turn down the volume of their busy minds and turn up their neurophysiological wellness. And after the first few sessions the practice becomes about their experience and not my explanations anyway.

Experienced teachers/facilitators have a personal repertoire of pedagogical "moves" that work, that they are comfortable engaging with and that provide the desired outcomes of the learning objectives. Novice teacher/facilitators are often uncertain what works and with whom and what expectations their organizations have regarding outputs and participant engagement. The goal of Yogic Peace Education (yogic peacebuilding) is not to perfect your curriculum or specialize your pedagogy but to foster a learning environment that is engaged, positive, responsive and beneficial. As has been said in other places, "it's not a doing, it's an undoing!"

Six. Learning Peace

Preparing for Change

There are many preparatory exercises that we can engage in as potential yogic peacebuilders. As "the learning process in peace education is understood primarily as experiential and activity-based rather than, for instance, learning by rote memorization or learning by repetitive conditioning" (Synott, 2006, 12), and while Yoga and peace education have compatible epistemological (nature of knowledge) and ontological (nature of the existence) underpinnings, Yogic Peace Education considers three vital preconditions to this activity-based practice: be safe, be curious (open-minded), and be respectful. Not all persons will come to this practice from the same place. Indeed, none of us has walked the same pathway to get here nor will we each walk forward in the same direction and, in instances where the yogic peace educator cannot provide safety, approach peacebuilding from a place free of prejudice or permit spaces for personalization of the practice, it may be suitable to delay communicating the discipline until these important qualities are present.

Prior to the deployment of any of the Yogic Peace Education techniques discussed later in this book, we advocate two imperative requirements:

1. Before connectivity with others the yogic peacebuilder must take the time to tune in (be present), evoke a wellness intention (choose to act as an instrument of wellness) and pledge to treat others with thoughtful kindness (this is a vital component of yogic peace pedagogy).
2. Prior to learning yogic peace education the following preparatory exercises are recommended for novice student/ teachers.

During preparatory exercises, a teacher/peacebuilder can observe the capacity of each student and ensure that the techniques are experienced as calming and integrating, rather than distressful and psychologically overwhelming. Some of the preparatory exercises are taught in the classroom while others are aspects of the student's individual lifestyle choices. These exercises develop the capacity for reflection, awareness, *ahimsa* and sensitivity within the peace practitioner.

Preparatory Techniques

1. Therapeutic Journaling
2. Sensory modulation
3. Emotional regulation
4. Preparatory breathing practices
5. The food we eat
6. Thoughts as thoughts only
7. Being with loss
8. Cultivating a natural loving response towards life
9. Smiling
10. Developing self-regulation

Many of the following exercises can be adapted to be used in the classroom and with community groups. However, we must be mindful that some of us may have experienced trauma or come from unstable countries, perhaps having directly experienced displacement, violence and tragedies. In these cases, exercises, that tune the mind to directly remember traumatic loss, may be experienced as overwhelming; they may potentially trigger psychological flooding and a deep dissociative state. In the worst scenario, they may trigger physiological reexperiencing and other traumatic symptoms. *It is important that students are encouraged to not go to their most traumatic loss in this instance.*[2] Those undergoing healing, involved with experiences of dislocation, trauma and distress, require careful attention. From the list above we begin with the most easily accessible integrating practice.

Written Expression

Written expression can be a worthwhile preparation for students about to be initiated into Yogic Peace Education techniques. It can allow a deeper processing so that other techniques are experienced as safe and secure. A brief written emotional expression task developed by Pennebaker and Beall (1986) had experimental participants write an essay expressing their feelings about a traumatic experience in their life (e.g., *write about your deepest thoughts and feelings about a particular incident*), whereas control participants were asked to write about innocuous topics (e.g., *write about your plans for the day*). This writing task was found to lead to significantly improved health outcomes in healthy participants. Change was not dependent upon writing about trauma but emerged from *writing in general*. Health was evidently enhanced in four areas: (i) reported physical health, (ii) psychological wellbeing, (iii) physiological functioning, and (iv) general functioning.

In addition to the physiological benefits from individual (and private) narrative expression, an advantage of this literary exercise is that one can use the language that one is the most expressive in. The following is an example of a written expression exercise. We suggest that both teacher and student allow time for the neural integration resulting from this exercise. Take your time—it is important that when you are engaged with written exercise therapy that you, as teacher or student, refrain from trying to make yourself feel better by engaging in activities or further therapeutic techniques such as energy work or visualization simultaneously. These techniques may be incorporated later in the teaching program.

Therapeutic Journaling
(Adapted from Pennebaker and Beall [1986])

1. Write for five minutes about your deepest thoughts and feelings about a painful experience. *Do not choose the most overwhelming experience that you have had.*
2. Do not censor your words or feelings. Write over the top of your words if you like. There is no intention to share or read over what you have written.
3. After you have written for the time period, destroy your writing.
4. Go for a walk or have plans to spend time with others.
5. Repeat this exercise for several days in a row.
6. Remember that you must write about both feelings and facts. If you only write about one of these (feelings or facts), there will be no integration or health improvement.
7. To begin with you may feel a deeper awareness of loss or inner discomfort. It is therefore important to follow steps 3 and 4.

As students engage with reflective writing processes, teachers/peacebuilders may also observe a greater interest and awareness of interconnections that transcend the purely intellectual. Kahane (2009) observed "a significant deepening of his students' interest in global justice issues and of understanding their implication in these issues after he engaged them in rigorous reflective observation of their bodily sensations and emotional patterns in response to their and others' suffering through the contemplative practices of meditation [and] free-writing" (Wong 2013, 279).

In such introspective processes, academic engagement with social justice loses its intellectual *himsa* of emotional dissociation—here circumstances are embodied reflectively instead of merely appreciated intellectually.

For the yogic peace educator written emotional expression can be a useful way of working within communities. It may be possible to facilitate the community to come together to write their shared narrative, again avoiding writing of the worst trauma.[3] The writing must include the facts of what happened and the feelings. Perhaps all those in the village or community can write their feelings and facts into the narrative. In some instances, this narrative can later be transformed into theatre or music (Boal 2000).

This process may also be extended into a vision for the future (Boulding 2000). For those in the community who are struggling to see any future vision of hope, it may be useful to encourage the voice of youth or children. It may be the young that can vision forward notions of peaceful community whereas mature individuals meet obstacles in imagining a different world.

Sensory Modulation

Sensory processing is the neurological process that organizes sensation from one's own body and the environment.

> Our primary connection with the physical world is through our body and its senses. When the overdominance of our discursive mind interferes with this connection, we objectify the world as separate from us, hence our emotional disassociation from it. [Bai] attributes the inertia that prevents us from taking action over the environmental disintegration and social injustice humanity is facing to our practice of education that is based on "disembodied ideas—ideas that are not worked into one's whole being with senses and feelings" [Bai cited in Wong 2013, 278].

Despite the fact that filtering out "bad" information using the intellect means we remain dislocated (and mentally *safe*) from many important experiences, we learn that we needn't be protected from the world around us once we increase our capacities to regulate our bodies' reactions to stimulus. Modulating our bodies' responses through the conscious use of the senses is a very useful skill to develop. Simple daily sensory modulation awareness provides useful solace when we experience discomfort from processing pain and trauma—so we don't need to ignore suffering but *change how we react* to suffering. As we develop a deeper *felt* engagement with the world around us we don't need to dislocate from others (and their experiences of violence and injustice). We need only to develop the capacity to *feel with others* by feeling with the whole self.

Sensory Modulation Self-Awareness Exercise
(Adapted from the Sensory modulation program [2015])

1. What is the difference between calming and alerting experiences?
2. Are there pros and cons to these two states?
3. Explore and identify what calms you.
4. Explore and identify what alerts you.
5. What kind of physical environments make you calm?
6. What kind of physical environments make you alert?
7. Explore how your feeling of calmness or alertness affects your emotions.
8. Explore how your feeling of calmness or alertness affects your communication style.
9. What kind of strategies can you identify that might assist you make healthy choices in the future?

We can use our senses (touch, taste, smell, vision, proprioception, and hearing) to *calm* or *alert* us according to our own preferences. For example, certain smells will be integrated by our nervous system as either deeply calming or powerfully alerting. If we develop awareness of our own preferences and sensory integration style, we can consciously utilize sensory experience to manage our reactions to our environment. This can be as simple as a hot bubble bath to calm, chewing a mint or cinnamon flavored gum to alert (maybe the smell of lavender works for you as calming or the smell of citrus is alerting—each of us needs to investigate our particular sensory experiences). As we use sense-strategies to enhance our wellness we can use our knowledge and self-awareness to manage our sensory responses. As our sensory awareness develops we may experience a deeper consciousness of an interconnectedness with others and their suffering.

Emotional Regulation

Emotional regulation can include a number of skills that assist you to be aware of your emotions, make plans to anticipate and regulate emotions that arise in difficulty, and notice how our emotions, thoughts and behaviors are all connected.

That said, the skill of emotional regulation on its own does not automatically lead to a peacebuilding personality. Through emotional regulation, knowledge has been found to moderate associations between personality traits and behavior. Côté, DeCelles, McCarthy, Van Kleef and Hideg (2015), in their experimental design with 131 participants, found a positive correlation between moral identity and prosocial behavior *but emotional regulation on its own was not significantly correlated with prosocial behavior*. In fact, this core facet of emotional intelligence was shown to promote both prosocial *and* interpersonally deviant behavior depending upon the moral identity of the participant.

Emotional Regulation Exercise
(Adapted from NYU *SOS for Emotion* Booklet [2016])

1. Define anger, joy, sadness, hurt and fear.
2. Where does stress come from?
3. How does stress feel?
4. Explore and identify a negative reaction to stress.
5. Explore and identify a positive response to stress.
6. What are *your* warning signs for distressful emotions?
7. What are some coping skills you use?
8. Can you think of any other coping skills?
9. What will it feel like the next time you feel stress?
10. What will you do the next time you feel stress?

The awareness of our capacity to feel, understand and modulate our emotional reactions to our environment is crucial when engaging with the suffering of others or entering traumatized communities. It is important in terms of managing our own responses to pain, deprivation and tragedy and is important in terms of the way in which we will begin to respond (a mindful action) rather than react (a mindless action). "Inner peace is necessary for political peace and justice because one cannot blindly go into action without understanding the social, cultural and political dimensions in which one experiences the world" (Wiggins 2011, 218).

We need inner composure or we cannot possibly engage with outer discord. Locating our own well of peace is a crucial first step in building peace.

Preparatory Breathing Techniques

Our nervous system is profoundly affected by our breathing. A range of yogic breathing practices have been developed which serve to modulate our senses and prepare our systems for embodied aspects of *ahimsa*. Breathing can lead to "inner self-confidence, purification and an enhanced ability to resolve conflicts and monitor aggression" (Jefferson-Buchanan 2006, 33). Mindful breathing helps control our thoughts and has been shown to calm verbal aggression, increase relaxation, and improve concentration, attention and vitality (Kauts and Sharma 2009). The simplest preparatory exercise is to observe our own breath.

Observing the Breath

1. Set an alarm for a certain time frame (5, 10, 15 minutes).
2. Sit comfortably with eyes closed.
3. Bring your attention to the full inhalation. Without any physical or psychological force. Simply observe. Notice the breath coming into the nostrils and travelling all the way down past the diaphragm to the belly.
4. Bring your attention to the full exhalation. Without any physical or psychological force. Simply observe. Notice the effect of the breath leaving the body. Notice the physical pathway.
5. Relax, stay calm as you observe (in time, there may be a glimpse of a subtler experience of inner expansion and connection).

BREATHING VS. *PRANAYAMA*

Breathing is the act of inhaling and exhaling. Pranayama, a core practice of Yogic Science, involves the building up of the life force within an individual's nervous system using breath—the control of breath, the suspension of breath and the elongation of breath. While pranayama uses breathing, not all breathing is pranayama. Crucial differences between basic breathing and pranayama are the slow quality of breath in pranayama practices and the assistance of the diaphragm to deeply breathe through the nostrils (Jerath et al. 2006). A main difference is that pranayama is mindful and intentional (often using ratio of in breath: out breath, counting duration and employing physical considerations that can include body position and breath retentions and extensions). There are a variety of pranayama techniques and many are used in Yoga classes to acquire, develop and sustain states of pranic wellbeing.

> Popular pranayama techniques include deep, even, three-part inhales and exhales, alternate nostril breathing, forceful expulsion of breath using the diaphragm and abdominal muscles, and slow diaphragmatic breathing with partial closure of the glottis creating an audible sound of rushing air described "like an ocean" [Gard et al. 2014, 4].

Merely beginning to become more aware of the breath is a pathway to greater neuro-physiobiological wellness. As you begin to notice the breath there is a movement away from "automatic" breathing to "mindful" breathing. We may feel many of our circumstances in life are out of our control, and indeed this is the truth for many moments in our life cycle, but in many instances you CAN control how you breathe. In instances where other options of Yogic Peace Education are not possible, one can still check-in with one's breathing and become an instrument of wellbeing.

Mindful Eating

According to Yogic Science the basis of life is the physical bodies of individuals. The quality of the body influences the quality of the mind. Within Yogic Science the physical body is formed from the quality and quantity of the food that is ingested:

> "*Annam*" means food and "*mayam*" means that which pervades completely. *Annamayam* is the outermost and grossest physical aspect of the individual's constitution. This aspect is available for the sense organs to perceive. It is named as "*annam*" since it is born out of food, sustained by food and is going to become food in the end. The earth part of the physical body will merge with the earth; the water portion will merge with water and so on [Chandrasekaran 2012, 64].

Physical food should be eaten slowly, with internal attitudes of gratitude and enjoyment. This allows the digestive system to function correctly. Yogic Science recommends the following:

> The norm recommended is half the stomach is for food, a quarter [of] the stomach for water and the remaining quarter for air. Appropriate food nourishes the body whereas inappropriate food brings destruction to the body [Chandrasekaran 2012, 65].

Yogic Science recognizes that *what* food is eaten also influences an individual's emotions and mind. It is therefore an important aspect of consideration and practice for any individual wishing to practice *ahimsa*, the natural, life nourishing mental stance. As Chandrasekaran (2012) states, "Mind stuff is also made from the essence of food. Therefore, food effects emotions. Inappropriate food pre-disposes one to physical, physiological and psychological disorders" (66).

Each individual has his or her own requirements and reactions to food. A diet that gives the most inner stability, strength and vitality is a platform for the development of *ahimsa*. In Yogic Science it is recognized that true progress is never forced and this is pertinent when developing a peaceful relationship with food. It is not possible to experience or embody peace if we remain in a fight with our body or mind. Additionally, what is suitable for one person may not hold true for another and this is particularly relevant at the physical level of development and maintenance. Inherent in this suitability is the temporal act of observing how food (and which food) affects us. So that it is not simply a matter of choosing but of observing the *outcome* of each choice.

Mindful Eating Exercise

1. Select a food that makes you feel stable, strong and vital.
2. Create an environment for eating that is free of distractions and clutter (turn off screens and sit comfortably).
3. Partake of a bite of this food and chew it slowly.
4. Take a moment to savor the food.
5. Swallow the food.
6. Investigate how you feel.
7. Do you feel nourished and satisfied or disturbed and unsatisfied?
8. Ask yourself if you desire to eat more of this food.
9. Eat more but stop when you imagine your belly is half full.

As you practice mindful eating you will cease to unconsciously fill your body with food that is inappropriate, un-nourishing or harmful. Investigating which foods are the best for you means taking control of your eating in such a way that each bite becomes a conscious decision and when you eat mindfully you also digest fully and contribute to the wellness of your human instrument.

THOUGHTS AS THOUGHTS ONLY

One of the key outcomes of yogic practice is an inhibition of negative appraisal, emotional reactivity and rumination. In this process individuals no longer identify themselves with thought but are able to observe inner mind activities from a distance. This capacity is of immense value in the development of a life-nourishing stance. Wong (2013) argues that this capacity is an important precursor in the development of critical reflective practice and leads to a conscious appreciation of what is transpiring in our minds.

> Very often we are run by habitual thoughts, most of which are ideas, ideologies, or "systemic chatter" (Hyles and Vinksy 2012) we have internalized from the systems or cultures we reside in. Our capacity to notice the mental chatter creates a pause between us and the thoughts with less identification, and hence the space needed for critical and reflective investigation into how we may be implicated in reproducing social injustice, and how we can creatively address relations of power [Wong 2013, 280].

Similar to other preparatory practices used in Yogic Peace Education, the practice of "thoughts as thoughts only" uses awareness to build up conscious understanding.

Thoughts as Thoughts Only Exercise

1. Wait until you are stimulated by something that enters your senses (this can be something you see, hear, feel, etc.)
2. Notice your unconscious (knee-jerk) response to what has occurred. Notice that your mind has a reaction to something you are sensing. Simply notice that you are having a reaction.
3. Do not attach any judgment to your thought reactions. Simply observe that your thoughts arise and "notice" them.
4. When your thoughts arise also notice that in a few seconds other thoughts arise.

The idea of thoughts as thoughts relates to the maxim that "nothing is needed in this moment" and that one can recognize that one can notice what is going on in one's head (body, life) without taking immediate action.

Being with Loss Without Avoidance

The simplest path out of pain and perpetual misery is to learn to sit with the discomfort or loss, merely sitting with the discomfort and waiting alongside it with our eyes closed. There is nothing to be done. Just sit and wait and then there is a shift in energy, a transformation. This is what compassion is. Later this occurs naturally when we sit quietly with others who are in pain. There are many versions of this most simple practice. The one included here encourages intention and observation.

Being with Loss Exercise
(Adapted from *The Little Book of Mindfulness*
by Patrizia Collard [London: Gaia Books, 2014, 63].)

1. Sit comfortably.
2. Focus on breathing. Take a natural full breath in and retain gently.
3. Focus on a loss. Perhaps it is a loss of health, friendship, partnership, country or even cherished belief system.
4. Very simply you can be with the loss through a simple statement of intention, "Let me feel the..." As the feeling of loss comes into your awareness, just sit with it. Do not judge it, do not blame and do not avoid. Simply breathe in gently and observe. Do not pretend that the pain is not there. As you breathe allow yourself to consciously relax. Wait for a minute or two and then return your awareness to the breath of life.

The yogic practice of *asana* can be translated from the Sanskrit to English as "to sit with." This is a major component of classical Yogic Science and this speaks to the importance in yogic practice of simply being (rather than doing). The practice of "sitting with" an emotion of loss is an active engagement of feeling that allows us to cultivate wellness in the wake of loss.

Cultivating an Automatic Loving Response Towards Life's Diversity

Lin (2006) uses the term "peace intelligence," which is "associated with a deep love for all lives, a deep compassion for all existences, a courage and conviction for unconditional forgiveness and reconciliation" (68). All yogic pathways—including Yogic Peace Education—contain processes that identify this as an outcome of sincere practice. Automatic loving is the result of an integrated, concentrated contemplation—meditation.

Simple *Metta* Meditation Exercise
(Adapted from *The Little Book of Mindfulness*,
by Patrizia Collard [London: Gaia Books, 2014, 82]).

1. Visualize emotional heat at the center of your chest.
2. Gently think the following intentions:
   May I be safe and protected
   May I be peaceful
   May I live at ease and with kindness
   May we be safe and protected
   May we be peaceful
   May we live at ease and with kindness
   May all beings be safe and protected
   May all beings be peaceful
   May all beings live at ease and with kindness

Metta is a Sanskrit word that can be translated as "loving kindness" and refers to practices of sending outward deep feelings of love to others. The previous exercise is a simple *metta* meditation that encourages such a mind-set (Collard 2014).

THE OPPOSITE OF FROWNING

According to research by Ekman, Davidson, and Frissen (1990) there are two classes of smiles. Genuine smiles of pleasure occur spontaneously during positive times together and involve the orbicularic muscle. Polite smiles do not involve this muscle. Genuine smiles come from within. To cultivate inner pleasure one can "practice" the art of smiling.

The Smiling Exercise

1. Shut your eyes.
2. Take a gentle breath in and a gentle breath out.
3. Bring your lips into a gentle smile.
4. Pause.
5. Observe the inner feeling of the smile.
6. Relax into this feeling, breathing gently all the while.

What is interesting is that people can predict a genuine smile and have changes in brain electromyography readings *before* they see another person's smile (Heerey and Crossley 2013). Social mimicking or responding does not trigger a natural or genuine smile; a genuine smile comes and creates true pleasure from within.

Developing Optimal Self-Regulation

Thus far, this book has explored ways that a peacebuilder could begin the necessary preparation for embodying the qualities of integrity, nonviolence, simplicity, spiritual connection, self-awareness and self-mastery from the perspective of Yogic Science. Yogic Science is applied and rests upon practices rather than ideas or words; it is not the reasons behind why something is effective often that contributes to change but the practice itself (Yogi Sri K. Pattahbi Jois famously maintained that Yoga is 99 percent practice and 1 percent theory). What follows is a description of the core practices for maintaining optimal self-regulation and balance in Yogic Science. The following practice comes from the program at the Rashtriya Sanskrit Vidyapeetha, India, as taught in 2012. This is the most challenging of all the preparatory exercises as it comes directly from Yogic Science. It may necessitate Yoga training or a Yoga instructor to administer.

Developing Self-Regulation Exercise

Begin the day at sunrise.

1. Move the bowels, wash the face and have a glass of water.
2. Tune the mind towards an attitude of gratitude towards the divine. This can involve the chanting of *sloka* (a passage taken directly from yogic philosophy), a prayer, or an inner attunement of some kind such as a mantra. This first action is usually done in the auspicious pose (*swasthikásana*) or easy pose, and is said to promote physical and mental stability while relieving any stiffness in the knees or joints. It is useful to have a pleasant facial expression.
3. Follow with introductory *pranayama*. Before practicing *pranayama* any imbalance such as excess body fat, mucus blockage, gas in the stomach and intestines, etc., should be

eliminated. We recommend that a qualified Yogic Science expert introduce the class to simple *pranayama* such as alternate nostril breathing (*nadi shodhana* or a*nulom vilom*). In the meantime, students may be taught the full yogic breath. Inhaling slowly, feel the abdomen expand first, then the chest, and finally feel the air filing the throat region. With the exhale, expel the air from the abdomen and then the chest. Ensure that students understand the difference between this practice of full yogic breath and abdominal breathing, where only the abdomen moves.

4. Salute to the sun (*Vaidika Surya Namaskara*) is the next daily practice (this is a physical activity described fully in many Yoga manuals and a qualified Yoga teacher can demonstrate/assist). This gives flexibility to the whole body, reduces fat around the hips, stomach and thighs and relieves laziness.

5. Rest in corpse pose (*shavasana*). Lying on your back with legs hip distance apart and palms facing upwards, allow your body to deeply relax and absorb the benefit of the salute to the sun series.

It is important to note that *pranayama* should be practiced in a pure (*sattvic*) state of mind. The proper practice of *pranayama* leads to health, while improper practice leads to illness (*Hatha Yoga Pradipika*, 2, 16). According to the *Hatha Yoga Pradipika*, holding breath in for brief periods can be of benefit, "by stopping the prana through retention, the mind becomes free from all modifications" (*Hatha Yoga Pradipika*, 2, 77). Beginner breath retention follows the ratio 1:4:2: inhale for one unit, hold for 4 units and exhale for 2 units (if you inhale for 4 beats, hold for 16 and exhale for 8). In *pranayama* (yogic breathing exercises) it is always advisable that students double the length of time it takes to breathe in when breathing out. Retention (*kumbhaka*) is best done with the supervision of a qualified Yoga pranayama teacher but incorporating it into your morning routine can reduce body inflammation and increase oxygenation (the Bohr Effect) of our human instrument.

> JANINE: When I began classes I thought I was flexible, especially when compared to others my age. So I was surprised and a little disappointed when my teacher asked me to practice only the salute to the sun series; many

repetitions of this series in the one class. I think this continued for six weeks. Slowly, slowly my body regulated itself and all pain and digestive issues normalized. I did not realize how much pain my body had taken for granted and no longer recognized. I was amazed at how such a simple process was able to create such change.

This series gives a stable and balanced start to the day. We note that there are many similarities to practices from other cultures, including the Muslim prayer series. The usefulness of this practice is not revealed in its intensity, but in its regular and systemized practice. When the body brings itself back into circulatory, digestive, muscular skeletal and nervous system health, it is possible to move into a full Yoga class. From this base a student may begin simple processes of concentration and meditation. It may be useful for us to state that this process is not exactly fun or enjoyable. Yet over time the fruits of a balanced neuro-psychobiological system reveal itself. Despite the commodified way in which Yoga has been introduced to the West, true change or optimal self-regulation does not come from momentary experiences of calmness or euphoria or pleasure.

KATERINA: I had done Kundalini Yoga before and it was mostly energizing postures with lots and lots of breath work and mantra work. I literally felt like it was designed for my body and had the sense that I had stumbled upon something that I could do well from the first day (cue the ego...). However, the first time I took a power Yoga class (I did not know at the time it was a Vinyasa class taken almost exclusively from the Ashtanga Primary Series) I was literally incapable of everything ... all of it was unsettling and most of it was impossible. Standing poses made me feel weak, seated poses left me confused and dizzy and the sun salute! Holy Shmoly! I remember my first Chaturanga Dandasana (what is commonly called plank position) as I went to step back (I was not jumping back no matter how many people around me bounced from the top to the bottom of their mats without effort) and when I achieved the start of the position (all of this by watching others in the monkey-see monkey-do method you are left with in large classes) I lasted half a second before dropping from the belly button like a stone! Ten years later I am still unpacking my sun salute but it has become my go-to practice on a daily basis.

The Yogic Peacebuilder

Peace educators are not necessarily yoginis (and vice versa). This volume, while inspired and infused with Yogic Science, does not confuse being yogic practitioners with teaching peace. The goal of Yogic Peace Education is to provide tangible materials and exercises that introduce practices conducive to outcomes similar to, or systemic in, the art and science of Yoga. As mentioned in previous sections, the goal of the practice manual is not to duplicate existing Yoga materials under the rubric of peace education; rather to corral the appropriate means and methods that a yogic peace educator would find useful. There are ample sources and suppliers of yogic knowledge and many fine teachers (should students wish to study the yogic path). This next section introduces a peace education peacebuilding tool kit inspired by yogic knowledge (see Figure 9). The toolkits take root from the five principles of Yogic Peace Education introduced in the beginning of Chapter 6. We recall these practices here:

FIGURE 9
Five Principles of Yogic Peace Education

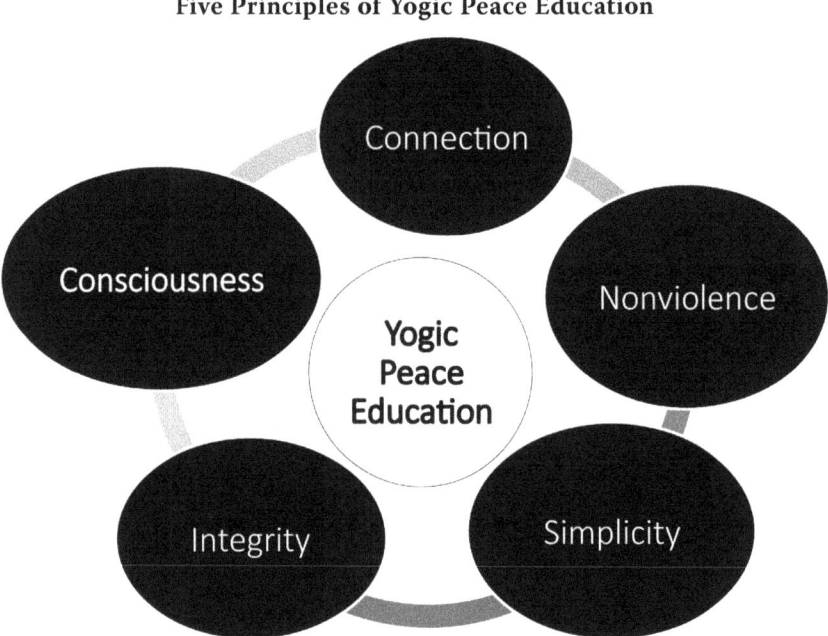

Toolkit 1: Learning Without Violence

Learning is the work of the human animal. We are learning beings and from the time we are born our existence is marked by what we have learned, how we learn to learn, what we want to learn, what we cannot seem to learn no matter how much we try, how we embody our learning and what learning we inevitably share with others. This aspect of living or life-long learning should not be confused with "having" something you give to somebody else; it is a gentle act of communicating experiences, wisdom and wonder as you cultivate experience and then share it with others.

You are made to learn—but learn what you may ask? In Yogic Peace Education the knowledge that is around you, that comes from the environment and your senses, is one kind of knowledge but the inner knowledge you gain by nurturing practices that allow you to voyage inward, produces a singular and ephemeral knowing that is particular to you and only you, in this moment (and in a moment there is change). Change is life, life is learning. If we allow our self-knowledge to be as important as (or more important than) that knowledge that comes from outside of ourselves, we begin to be able to fully engage with our intention to learn without violence.

1. Integrity

Learning without violence rests upon the idea that as human beings we are in a constant responsive relationship with the world around us. The words integrity and integrate have the same root: *wholeness*. Integrity (integration) practice means identifying that learning is not something separate from other parts of human experience (Stephenson 2012). At all moments we are learning. This is irrespective of our age or whether we perceive ourselves to be in a rut or not.

The **first integrity practice** is to acknowledge that you yourself are always shaping and being shaped by the forces around and within you (you are whole and connected to the whole universe). The **second integrity practice** is to understand that you always have a choice in terms of how learning experience unfolds within you. *Yes, always.* We know this seems unbelievable, but we do have this power once we decide it is so. **How, you ask?** You need to cultivate the practice of knowing that you have the capacity to make any experience in life playful, responsible and purposeful. When we take things in, learn things that are new, we integrate our learning. In many instances, in education, what you learn seems to be outside of you (classical banking education identified by Paolo Freire (2003)). But to imagine learning practices as external to your instrument means you perceive of the act of learning as an *acquisition*. This is not necessary. You can choose to look at learning in a manner wherein the act of learning is part of being human and that it is not *what you learn* or *the way you learn* (or your learning is measured) but the way you perceive of learning.

We are human so we are learning animals. We are thoughtful creatures so the mind has a great deal of influence on how we embody (integrate) information and how that knowledge impacts our physio-neurological selves. **Learning as an act of breathing.** You do not breathe competitively (generally, unless you are in a breath holding competition) so you do not need to learn in a competitive way either. You do not need to learn things simply to perceive that you are *more than* someone else and your ability to test well, or less well, does not mean you are *less than* someone else who learns something better. We are all learning all the time. Judging what you learn as more or less important is an exercise that inevitably just leads to feelings of inequality and separateness. This is sometimes quite hard in mainstream education where marks and grades and degrees and certificates are considered measures of us that are inevitably competitive. Yogic Peace Education considers this evaluation a form of violence. To learn without violence, we need to integrate the act of learning into our being and ignore, resist and contest the perception that the outcomes of education *increase* our humanity. They do not—neither do they diminish it. We are fully human with or without schooling. This integrity work allows you to stop comparing, to relax and develop your own awareness of incorporating internal and external information into knowledge. Learning is not something that we copy or duplicate into our minds but something that we naturally step into and incorporate into our whole being.

Integrity Practice
1. Ask yourself what it means to learn something?
2. Ask yourself what motivates you to learn something?
3. Ask yourself what it feels like to succeed at learning?
4. Ask yourself what it feels like to *not* succeed at learning?
5. When was the first time you learned something?
6. What was the last thing you learned?
7. Take a moment and try to recollect a time you were with someone else when they were learning something. What did you feel being present when someone else was learning? Were you frustrated? Delighted? Surprised? Happy?

Six. Learning Peace

For many parents reading this, the joy of a child "learning" how to crack an egg into a bowl when making cookies or "learning" how to zip up a jacket when going outside becomes an undertaking of independence, a sign of development and an action of pleasure. The goal of integrity practice is to consider all human acts and experience as learning moments.

> KATERINA: Since elementary school I avoided subjects in school where I had obstacles to getting good grades. I suffered from dyslexia as a young child and it showed itself in both letters and numbers. I literally cannot write a word beginning with "s" to this day without writing the rest of word first and going back and then adding the "s" (if writing "stop" I would hand write "top" then add the "s"!). After a summer school teacher found out about my condition, she helped me find strategies to overcome my learning disability. Afterward, I was able to work with letters but numbers still mostly eluded me. I always thought of myself as someone stuck in a world without numbers and considered this made me deficient in some way. Algebra? No way. Statistics? Forget it. What I didn't realize at the time was that my ability to learn around my perceptions was the real key to loving my learning. It was not that I was or was not GOOD at something but that I found areas where my learning was a delight. I learned the act of learning was everywhere, in every day, that sometimes I had to learn the same thing over and over (don't step into a cold shower) and that does not make me any less worthy.
>
> JANINE: The week before my exams was a difficult time and unusual for me as for some reason I could not remember or even memorise any of the material. I was upset as I realized that I wanted to honor my teachers by doing well and yet it seemed as if my brain would not cooperate. In the end I remember just surrendering inside myself. I trusted that there was something that I was being taught and that I could trust this process also. I chose to go into the exams without any fear, totally relaxed, with a sense of inner lightness. There was no feeling of wanting to achieve well or even distress that I was going to fail. In each exam I found myself sitting quietly with each question. Inside myself the knowledge would come forward and I would write the words down. In the questions for management of health issues, the faces of different people that I loved would come forward in my mind's eye and I would see the ways that Yoga therapy could assist them. I could also see how the disease was formed and maintained in their body. It seemed so natural that I was not even aware that this happened until I reflected many months afterwards. I achieved distinction in this postgraduate diploma. But more than this I was gifted an experience of faith and willingness to be guided by life.

2. NONVIOLENCE

Bring into your awareness the intention that you will embrace a perspective of life affirmation and life nourishment in all your words, thoughts and deeds. **From this point on, *on this day,* until you go to sleep, you will engage with both inner and outer information from a positive, protective and supportive place.** Think it's easy? Try ... notice how quickly negative thoughts arise when you are in the active place of learning, be aware of thoughts that lead to anxiety, fear, dissatisfaction, inequality and depression. Notice how the mind jumps to "bad" places so easily; how it comes to compare and judge and differentiate everything.

In this nonviolence practice *be different to what you have been.* Be positive, happy, delighted, even. And then notice something else—in your curiosity see how this flows *easily and naturally* from you. Once you take on a positive stance it becomes easier to maintain it. Cracking the egg is challenging, the first step feels like something is broken. All is good. Be aware you may re-learn what you discover over and over again; re-learning is part of learning. Be okay with that. Accept it. Relax into this possibility.

If this nonviolent practice does not resonate for you, rest easily with your own intention and try something else. Be flexible and creative. Move the word "violence" away from your lexicon, bring your mind into awareness of other possibilities and ways of relating, other options, words, possibilities. Perhaps you may choose to limit the amount of second hand violence you receive into your system.

Perhaps you will choose to work in communities with issues of poverty, global and/or local violence. Perhaps you are already living in these communities. If so, attune your mind to the possibilities within the situation in a new manner. Tune your mind to hope within the chaos. *Light your personal candle and see how far the light goes.* It is not easy but protect your flame at all costs. Take small practical steps to improve the situation; courage breeds hope. Hope brings inspiration. Inspiration brings transformation.

3. Simplicity

Start each day with the intention that you will learn easily without any force or distress within your neuro-psycho-physiological-spiritual system. Observe fear based conditioning in relation to learning and understand it makes things very complicated. Simple is best. Do not require a mental conditioning but rather, breathe easy, rest and watch these "ways of knowing" dissolve. Allow yourself to feel gratitude and joy at the privilege of being able to learn in a different way. Walk away from your mind and simply breathe and smile into your life.

4. CONNECTION

Remembering that you have a spiritual dimension, that you are not separated from anything else, is the first step in developing awareness. It is not *out there*, it is not external, not an "othering" accessed through psychic means. It is simply recognition that unity is the nature of all things. Separation is the illusion we are convinced comprises reality. It is not true. The opening of awareness confirms the connectivity of all things and this subtle intelligence is something that you can relax into because *it is you*.

Let go of notions of separateness and, as you relax into unity, you will become aware of any limiting conditioning that has been imposed upon you through fear and distress. Then, you can observe patterns of avoidance that used to protect you and dismantle them to craft yourself gently in a different way. You are free to deepen your inner silence and transform away from violence. It is not something others need to see; it is not something that you *represent*; it just is. This can be the natural work of a lifetime. It becomes a way of attuning your cognitive self; moment by moment, second by second, until it is natural to you.

Connection Practice
1. Imagine how you are separate from the people around you.
2. Imagine what stands between you (between you and the person next to you, the tree beside you, the ground underneath you).
3. How do you feel?
4. Now imagine you are connected to the people around you.
5. Imagine that all things that surround you are connected to you.
6. How do you feel?

The previous exercise comes from another person's imagination, yet you may find it enjoyable. You may find that you have a glimpse of the wellness that is innate within you. While the benefits are described in concrete terms, remember that your nervous system, your neuro-psychobiological-spiritual system is unique. This practice may suit you or it may not. It may suit you some days but not others. Listen to your own inner sense of what is soothing and nourishing for you at this time. Unblocking of energy is not the goal. Sometimes the blockages are useful and necessary. *Conceiving of yourself as "blocked" in some way is not useful.* So relax and let it be natural. Often the simple practices of sitting still, quiet and connected are all that is necessary.

5. Consciousness

Can you live inside your own body-mind system without negative or positive judgment? Can we? Can I? Gandhian peace education (of which Yogic Peace Education is an example) considers this the first call to peace. Can we live inside a body-mind system that is subject to racism and prejudice and not be that? Can we be free of the hate that is projected onto us from the outside? Can we?

Can we accept our own pain, and insecurities with compassion, humor and love? Can we do this without devaluing the ways that we have earned these scars? Can we do this without covering up the atrocities that are being committed daily on the environment, the planet and on all living forms of life? Can we express ourselves in a way that is revolutionary without feeding on hate, despair and fear, or conduct ourselves without consciously comparing our suffering to the suffering of others? Can we step away from the implicit historical grudges held within our religious organizations or our cultural groups? Can we step away from the conditioning of our ancestors, our genders, and our social groups? Gandhi found his own way of doing this but can we help each other learn how to do this too? Perhaps. Inevitably we each find our own way, individually or collectively, to do this. **Conscious self-awareness sees the whole picture while rising above it—cultivate awareness, integrate with consciousness and then breathe and let go.** Self-awareness practice is not about controlling or directing something within your nature but about becoming aware of existence, then ceasing to feel that understanding means we are somehow in a position of authority or domination because of what we have learned. Despite what we learn we do not have (nor are we expected to have) all the answers—we encourage the journey—question and enjoy the quest.

Toolkit 2: Living Without Violence

Living completely without violence is not straightforward, and despite the fact that living completely without violence is probably impossible (to live you must eat and to eat living things means there is violence) throughout this book we have argued that it is possible to embrace a life-nourishing perspective to minimize harm. The life-nourishing mindset is nurtured by simplicity, time with nature, gratitude, faith and joy. One systematically clears any fear based psychological reactions and simply observes without inner physiological stir. It is not an invitation to do nothing but an invitation to begin to understand that sometimes action is *not* required. Often a life nourishing perspective is implicitly political and radical and sometimes it can be drastically simplistic (radical love means exactly that—to love as an act of profound action). Our choices create our communities. Our choices contribute to our circumstances. Our choices generate our inner experiences of outer stimuli. Our choices, when we exercise them consciously, are immensely powerful.

1. INTEGRITY

Integrity is the quality of being whole and undivided; or the quality of being honest and having strong moral principles. Integrity practice as we view it, is the process of maintaining a certain inner awareness towards developing and maintaining non-fear based thought and action. While this seems philosophical, it is not; it is a practical process of growing your own inner conscience and morality (=integrity). It is not a belief system or rules imposed on you by others but a natural aspect of living. Each moment life gives opportunities to express and develop inner attunement. It is natural, i.e., a humanization of the system contents into the life's.

At a yogic level **the first integrity practice** is the use of the will to set the intention that at all times one is true to the practice of *ahimsa*. It is done from an inner condition of relaxed silent awareness and faith; a simple attunement at the start of each day.

Integrity Practice
1. Strip yourself of what you think you know and what you think you don't know (empty your assessment tank!).

2. Ask yourself what is experientially true for you.
3. Do you value nonviolence?
4. Does it resonate for you? *If it does not then do not pretend that it does.* Sit quietly and see what is within you.
5. What motivates you?
6. Is peacebuilding a desire to help others?
7. Is it a desire to be seen as a good person?
8. What is more important to being a peacebuilder: thoughts, words or deeds? Why?
9. Free yourself from any judgments about your desires and assumptions. Just notice what is.

Allow the development of your own authenticity in its own time and find your own intuitive responses to life where they are today. Let your integrity practice rest lightly on your shoulders as neither profound nor superficial. Let it be responsive to your own intuitive intelligence in this moment. Allow yourself to move away from defining things as good or bad (or yourself as good or bad) as you are neither good nor bad. You just are—things just are—people just are. This is potentially a space or inner perspective that allows humor, joy, collaboration and the capacity to build bridges to one other.

And there is nothing to avoid here. You are free to liberate yourself from limiting judgment and assumption. Remember that your thoughts are coming from limited data, limited knowledge and it is easy to get lost in your own thought processes (a pathway of identity that makes us feel separated all over again). The formation of identity in Yogic Peace Education is a process of recognizing separation and then investigating the option of perceiving unity instead. But start where you are and just be there.

2. Nonviolence

Nonviolence in word, thought and deed is a practice that is private to each individual (who knows what a person is thinking!). As we conceive of nonviolence, it is a process of sharpening your attention towards the practice or knowledge of nonviolence as a default setting (to use a mechanistic term). Take a second and sense your current mentality (your current default setting): is it restful? Anticipating something? Crouching? Bored? The environment influences the contents of your mind but part of that environment is *how* your mind processes what comes into it from your sensory system. As you know, your senses are always ingathering information from your surroundings, related to all kinds of material including images, temperatures, hazards, hunger, other peoples' words, faces, needs—the list is endless. So in a sense, establishing nonviolence becomes a process of being at ease with the nature of the mind (how your mind accepts sensory information) not limiting or controlling what kind of information is gathered. *Ever tried to not think of something?* It quickly becomes the only thing you think about! So the goal is not to control or censor the mind but understand its nature.

Also, your mind is not you—your mind is a part of you that works to observe and make sense of the world around you but you are not a product of your mind. As you come to recognize that, you can actively step in and alter how your mind works. By recognizing how it functions, you cease to identify *your mind* with *your identity*—this is wonderfully freeing! If we are not our thoughts then we can release ourselves from the power of damaging memories, emotions and imagination and BE otherwise.

The goal is to create an inner distance through awareness; eyes open, heart open and without creating an inner reaction or judgment towards the contents of your mind (no physiological stir, no disturbance). Know your life but do not be disrupted by it. Become the watcher within. Ask yourself: what is going on in my mind? What are my typical responses to stimulus? What if I don't do what is typical next time? What happened when I did that? What happens if I do nothing next time and simply perceive what is happening? What if nothing is required of me? Can I do nothing? Is that allowed? In this emerging state of mind-awareness compassion, grace and awareness develops within you gently without effort. We cease to process everything around us simultaneously in a big flutter and from this place of calm awareness things come in but they do not ripple the water. It is an ongoing effort (and focus) to understand how the minds works. You falter, find the path again, falter again and continue so that you investigate your existence and then naturally walk the appropriate path for your nature.

Nonviolence Practice
1. What does being a "wonderful" human being mean?
2. What is wonderful about being human?
3. Sit quietly.
4. How could you manifest "wonderful" in your life?
5. Take a big breath in.
6. Repeat.
7. Take a walk.
8. Become aware of the life of the earth.
9. As you walk stay connected to what is around you.

Consciousness is the highest expression of nonviolence. To be in a state of intelligent, sensitive connection with your internal and external environment is to fully integrate your being with life nourishingness. Try. It is possible in any environment; day or night, rural or urban, alone or surrounded by multitudes of people. Try.

3. SIMPLICITY

Simplicity is the condition or quality of being plain and uncomplicated in form and design. Simplicity practices are limited only by your imagination, dedication, awareness and insight. For example: eating with presence and awareness often leads to an experience of simple joy and gratitude. Sitting and acknowledging the efforts of the sun, the farmers, factory staff and the planet itself, prior to eating, sends a simple message of gratitude. This simplicity practice creates natural changes within the practitioner. Over time these momentary experiences of simplicity become the norm. A simple mind is not overly complicated by future worry because it is active in the present tense; what is actually happening in this moment. This is a radical notion in our modern world. A simple perspective knows that all needs are met in a way that engenders a greater balance than one human can perceive. It is a quantum experience of self. It involves tremendous trust not to be concerned about the future and live in balance in the present moment. It involves nurturing a consciousness that allows you to live fully. Living fully means living in a way that resonates with your own values and integrity; no two lives have the same needs (or the same needs throughout the life cycle for that matter) and this means we cannot know our needs if we do not investigate them. Needs change. Figure out what is needed now. In many instances we think we need things that are actually not at all necessary to the art of living. It can be daunting to choose things that conflict with what others want us to choose. It can mean sticking out and then, just when everyone has put you into a category (oh Martin doesn't eat broccoli), making new choices when the time is right for you. This can often involve courage that comes from collaborating with like-minded community and may involve simultaneously engaging and disengaging from the systems around you. Being flexible with yourself also allows you to be flexible with others around you—your kids, your spouse, your friends and family. Honor what is happening right now. It is not something that another person can decide for you. You must look for what you need. No one can do it for you.

Simplicity Practice

1. Close your eyes.
2. Take a couple of deep breaths.
3. What do you want in this moment?
4. What do you need in this moment?
5. What do you not need?
6. Is there something you would like to give up?
7. Let it go.
8. Repeat.

> KATERINA: When I was 17 I became a vegetarian and shunned eating meat for twelve years. I did not have great health during this time and although I felt morally and ethically fortified my body was often weak and I fought cravings for sugary foods day and night. Many women vegetarians need milk products or meat products when pregnant or lactating and it has become normal for women to "listen to their bodies" during the act of bringing forth new life into the world. I wasn't pregnant when I ordered a non-vegetarian meal for the first time in twelve years, but I had spent six months practicing Kundalini Yoga (a practice that supports vegetarianism). What happened to me is that I had cultivated my inner ears and was finally able to "listen to my body" and my body was saying "eat meat." So I did and I continue to do so today. Despite the ideas that it is more sattvic to avoid animal products and disturbing foods—for me—eating meat was a simple choice that made me healthier. It is not a choice others made for me. I made if for myself.

JANINE: When I was younger and choosing not to eat meat it was such a difficult thing. My parents were concerned that it would affect my health. People were stressed because they felt I was criticizing their cooking and food choices. They worried about what to prepare for me to eat. Somehow it was polarizing. The exercising of my choice in this area was somehow radical. Certainly it was inconvenient. Yet in Yoga at certain stages of development the diet is limited but generally it is about when we eat, our attitudes during eating and how much we eat. Not too much or too little, no extremes. Not so much about whether to eat meat or not. The only limit that my teachers have consistently shared is to not drink alcohol.

In my research, listening to Raja Yoga practitioners from 36 different countries, it seemed that vegetarianism became a natural way of eating. They did not seem to have made a conscious decision about it, rather it just gradually happened. Somehow the desire for meat dropped away. I have experienced decades without the desire for meat. I have also had times, during extreme health events, where my body has urgently needed huge amounts of protein via lentils and anything else I could find (preeclampsia in pregnancy). I suspect that our bodies know what is required and when.

4. CONNECTION

What does it mean to be spiritual? Human beings have been concerned about the unseen dimensions of their experiences for a long time. Recently, in the field of health science, researchers asked ordinary people about their experience of spirituality. A meta-review of spirituality studies in the health sciences defines human beings' spiritual experiences as beyond organizational membership and comprised of: (i) an inner existential awareness, (ii) connection, (iii) energy or power, and (iv) transcendental experience (Chui et al. 2004). Schmidt-Wilk (2000) extends this definition by suggesting categories of "applied spirituality" and "pure spirituality." Pure spirituality was a "silent, unbounded, inner experience of pure awareness" (Heaton et al. 2004, 63) while applied spirituality referred to the practical applications and measurable outcomes that arose from the inner experience. De Jager Meezenbroek, Garssen, van den Berg, van Dierendonck, Visser and Schaufeli (2012) reviewed various spirituality questionnaires as tools for measuring spirituality as a universal human experience. They found that current questionnaires were inadequate for identifying a comprehensive understanding of the role of spirituality as a universal human experience, particularly as questions tended to be about specific belief systems or religiosity. "In view of this, we have defined spirituality as one's striving for and experience of connection with oneself, connectedness with others and nature and connectedness with the transcendent" (de Jager Meezenbroek et al. 2012, 338).

Connection Practice
1. Close your eyes.
2. Breathe.
3. Connect with yourself.
4. Breathe.
5. Connect with the people around you that you cannot see.
6. Breathe.
7. Connect with the people you love although they are not there.
8. Breathe.
9. Connect with the earth even if it is under the floor or building beneath you.
10. Breathe.
11. Connect with the sky even if it is above the roof or building above you.
12. Breathe.
13. Trace the connection from yourself, to your loved ones, to the earth and to the sky.
14. Stay connected.
15. Breathe.
16. Open your eyes.

5. Consciousness

The following routine is provided as a classical example of yogic lifestyle and, although it should be viewed as a modern day practice with deep cultural roots, we are reminded that such orthodox practices are not for everyone. As is mentioned elsewhere in this volume, there is no single lifestyle suitable for all persons and the presented lifestyle practices of *Sahaj Marg* demonstrate one tradition that seeks to give attention to an integrated range of lifestyle changes. The changes impact the physiology, psychology and spirituality of the individual and the nonviolent mastery of self-benefits from a change in attunement impact on all levels of our being.

One modern (established 100 years ago) Raja Yoga school, *Sahaj Marg*, integrates *yamas* (yogic restraints) and *niyamas* (yogic observances) into the following lifestyle practices or maxims (see Table 5). Practice of any of these maxims are said to positively lead to the expression of the other values.

Table 5 *Sahaj Marg* Ten Maxims

Maxim	Description of the Practice
1	Rise before dawn. Offer your prayer and puja (worship) at a fixed hour, preferably before sunrise, sitting in one and the same pose. Have a separate place and seat for worship. Purity of mind and body should be specially adhered to.
2	Begin your puja with a prayer for spiritual elevation, with a heart full of love and devotion.
3	Fix your goal, which should be complete oneness with God. Rest not till the ideal is achieved.
4	Be plain and simple to be identical with Nature.
5	Be truthful. Take miseries as divine blessings for your own good and be grateful.
6	Know all people as thy brethren and treat them as such.
7	Be not revengeful for the wrongs done by others. Take them with gratitude as heavenly gifts.
8	Be happy to eat in constant divine thought whatever you get, with due regard to honest and pious earnings.
9	Mold your living so as to rouse a feeling of love and piety in others.
10	At bedtime, feeling the presence of God, repent for the wrongs committed. Beg forgiveness in a supplicant mood, resolving not to allow repetition of the same (Source: Ram Chandra 1991).

Toolkit 3: Loving Without Violence

From a yogic perspective love is defined as a forceless dynamism that flows through everything, without which there is no life. From this perspective we are each a container through which love flows. It is the forceless energy that animates us and that is transformed into the physical world through our activities, through our relationships, through our words and through our thoughts. Loving without violence asks whether we can become a neuro-psychobiological-spiritual container which is life nourishing and mindful.

You are an instrument of love (this does not mean you have to immediately hug the person sitting next to you on the bus or instantly go out and pet kittens) and, because loving is a part of your human nature, you needn't avoid, manage or go without love. Love is energy. Love is the forceless force. Love is life.

1. INTEGRITY

As we realize ourselves as sophisticated neuro-psychobiological-spiritual containers through which the forceless force flows, there is an opportunity to gently dissolve the hold of the ego based personality—the I in everything—and see ourselves, and all things, as matter and energy. This sounds uncomfortable—you probably spent a lot of time figuring out who "you" are—how *you* like your hair, what toothpaste *you* use, the way *you* make (or don't) *your* bed. But it is a way to feel natural joy.

Integrity Practice
1. Close your eyes.
2. Imagine someone you love.
3. Notice how that makes you feel.
4. Imagine someone you dislike.
5. Notice how that makes you feel.
6. Now imagine that person you dislike and send them love.
7. Notice how it makes you feel.

2. NONVIOLENCE

Loving without violence means being aware of how our relationships with ourselves, our bodies and others *really* are. Do we say we love ourselves but choose poor foods to eat or rely on stimulants to get through the day, depressants to find rest? Do we say we love ourselves but repeat negative mental sentences to ourselves that keep us in a hurtful place? Do we love others without violence? Are we violently loved?

There is a difficulty for many of us to separate *passion* from violence. In many ways strong feelings make us and others feel very special. This is not abnormal. The techniques presented in this volume thus far all maintain the importance of seeing what is really there, being aware and calm in the face of information. This does not mean you love less; rather that your capacity to love is not "special" or contingent but boundless and restorative.

Nonviolence Practice
1. Close your eyes.
2. Think of something you care about.
3. Capture the image of that something and see yourself caring for that something lovingly.
4. Does the act of caring make you feel whole or fragmented?
5. Imagine yourself now. Imagine caring for yourself.
6. Capture an image of caring for yourself and stay with it for a moment.
7. How does that make you feel?
8. Breathe in.
9. Relax.
10. Let yourself have a moment of uncluttered intelligence.
11. Open your eyes.

3. Simplicity

The easiest thing to do is do nothing, right? Not exactly. For many people doing nothing is the hardest thing in the world to do. There is a constant feeling of "not enough," or "not good enough," running through our minds. Why? Look at the bestseller lists: there are few calls in the modern age to: *Complicate your life! Make things more difficult! Get busier and far less effective! Top 10 ways to get **more** chaos into your day!* There is a reason for this. Simplicity, taking things away from your to-do list, learning to sleep, to relax, to rest are practices that speak to the core of what it means to be human—humans are not brains on sticks. In more and more ways we are finding the mind-body-spirit connection to be in a constant state of panic (hormonally, chemically and physically). We take vacations for a reason. We unplug (or try to unplug) while we sleep so we can slow down the consistent deluge of external stuff so our bodies can rest. But many of us are not resting well and we wake to the impatient hoards between our ears. This simplicity practice is all about cultivating the practices of restoration.

Simplicity Practice
1. Dress warmly and lie down.
2. Be comfortable (if necessary pillows under your knees, softness beneath you, extra blankets or turning up the heat in the room).
3. Your eyes can be open or closed.
4. Relax.
5. Place your hands on your belly.
6. Take 8 deep breaths. Breathe bottom to top—into your belly first, then your chest and then your throat and then exhale from top to bottom.
7. Relax.
8. Breathe easy, naturally, when you need to.
9. Let yourself rest and observe your breath.
10. Rise when you feel it is time.

4. Connection

This may be the easiest practice in the entire volume. You are already connected. It is natural. The *idea* that you are disconnected is a form of conditioning. The *idea* that you have to seek spirituality is nonsense. You are alive—therefore you are spiritual. If you are breathing you live in a spiritual and connected world. So relax.

5. Consciousness

The final practice presented in this book can be used in place of any other practice. Loving without violence starts with you. It starts with how you understand love (it is the life force remember) and that you appreciate the innate integral nature of love. Conscious self-awareness practice for loving without violence is unnecessary as there is nothing to master or become aware of here that you do not already intrinsically know. Loving without violence asks us to make a gentle inquiry that can be used at any time, in any circumstances.

Consciousness Practice
1. Breathe in deeply.
2. Breathe out fully.
3. Rest.
4. Breath in deeply and hold the breath without struggle (relax the throat) for a time suitable to you.
5. Let go the breath.
6. Breathe easy.
7. Ask yourself what is needed in this moment?
8. Allow yourself to feel the love that is in you, of you and that surrounds you.
9. Rest, relax.
10. You really don't need to do anything special.
11. Breathe.
12. Smile.
13. Be.

Conclusions

Yogic Peace Education is a theory and practice manual that does not seek to prescribe or define *the* way forward but *a* way forward. Counterintuitively for many of us, this means a going *backwards*, to what we know to be true already and need to acknowledge once more. We, the authors of this book hope that in this ambiguity there is a deep respectful confidence in your ability to access your own inner integrity, your own inner nonviolence, your own inner simplicity, your own spiritual connectivity and your own conscious self-awareness.

In many ways this book is a manual of self-investigation that can be shared. This was one of our goals. We wanted a way for readers to repeatedly "check in" with themselves so that the practices became habits and the habits displaced actions, mindsets and opinions that lead to violence. We are not violent beings, our nature is not to hurt and be hurt. We can live otherwise. This book seeks to remind us what we already know, learning, living and loving without violence is the natural way.

For some of us this book is a reminder whereas for others this information is new and welcome. We hope that in exploring this book the Yogic Peace Education reader/teacher/peacebuilders have become more clear about methods to manage your own sense organs, your own mind and your own nervous systems. We hope that building peace and teaching peace changes *who* we are, not just what we think about and communicate. We hope that dimensions of inner perception have been glimpsed along the way and we urge you to share these practices with others after all, we are none of us fully human without each other.

Om Shanti (Peace).

Glossary

Ahimsa non-harming, non-hurting; ethical principle on the first limb of the 8-Limb path

Aparigraha greedlessness, non-acquisitiveness; ethical principle on the first limb of the 8-Limb path

Asana physical postures in Yoga; third limb of the 8-limb path

Ashram retreat or monastic community

Ash-tanga the 8-limb path provided in Patanjali's *Yoga Sutras*

Asteya nonstealing; ethical principle on the first limb of the 8-Limb path

***Bhakti* Yoga** yogic practice utilizing devotion

Bija means seed, the sound or vibration that resonates with a particular chakra (used in *mantra* practice)

Brahmacharya moderation; ethical principle on the first limb of the 8-Limb path

Chakras wheels of energy vortices that line the spinal energetic channel (*sushumna*)

Citta combination of both the energetic and physical bodies in Yoga metaphysics

Compassion love

Conflict discord, unease

Cultural Nonviolence nonviolence based upon a world view

Cultural Violence violence based upon a world view

Culture a shared, socially transmitted system of meaning

Dharana concentration, focus; sixth limb of the 8-limb path

Dhyana absorption, immersion; seventh limb of the 8-limb path

Glossary

Education   organized learning

8-limb path   English for *Ash* (eight) *Tanga* (limb) referring to Patanjali's 8-limb path described in the *Yoga Sutras.*

Empathy   understanding the feelings of others

Hatha Yoga   yogic practice combining *asana* and *pranayama*

Ishwara pranidhana   contemplating divinity or cosmic consciousness; ethical principle on the second limb of the 8-limb path

Jnana Yoga   yogic practice utilizing study

Karma Yoga   yogic practice utilizing service to others

Kriyas   yogic hygiene

Manas   receptor of sensory information, mind

Mandiram   place to do Yoga

Mantra   repetition of a syllable or phrase (often in Sanskrit) either vocally or using an inner silent voice (*Dharana* technique used to focus the senses and calm the mind)

Meditation   techniques that concentrate the senses to attain inner consciousness of our essential nature

Metta   kindness

Mindfulness   meditation technique of contemplation and awareness each moment

Mudras   yogic gestures

Negative peace   said to exist in a space free from overt (direct) violence

Niyama   observances in yogic science; second limb of the 8-limb path

Nonviolence   principle or practice of eschewing violence

Pacifism   principle or practice of eschewing violence; resistance to war

Peace education   organized learning that reduces or prevents violence and contributes to positive peace

Peace pedagogy   teaching that utilizes nonviolence and peace-learning

Peacebuilding   interventions that increase peace and inhibit violence

Peacekeeping   military maintenance of negative peace

Peacemaking   creating peace agreements between conflict parties

Positive peace   presence of symbiosis and equity in human relations

Prana   vitality, life force, energy

Pranayama   yogic breathing; fourth limb of the 8-limb path

Praxis   theory and practice leading to action

Raja Yoga "king's" Yoga, classical Yoga, Patanjali's 8-limb path

Samadhi bliss; eighth limb of the 8-limb path

Santosha contentment; ethical principle on second limb of the 8-limb path

Satya truthfulness, nonlying; ethical principle on first limb of the 8-limb path

Saucha cleanliness, purity; ethical principle on second limb of the 8-limb path

Shavasana corpse pose; supine position for the practice of letting go (death)

Surya Namaskar salute to the sun: vinyasa used in classical Yoga

Sushumna energetic channel that links the chakras

Swadhyaya self-study; ethical principle on second limb of the 8-limb path

Tapas "burning" up obstacles; seriousness; ethical principle on second limb of the 8-limb path

Vinyasa a series of postures in yogic asana practice

Violence deliberate and avoidable harm done to self or others

Yama restraints in yogic science; first limb of the 8-limb path

Yantra yogic images

Yoga to join, yoke, unify; technique used in personal transformation

Yogi male Yoga practitioner

Yogin Yoga practitioner

Yogini female Yoga practitioner

Appendix: Chakra Coloring Meditation

Original chakra coloring pages illustrated by Corey Standish

Coloring combined with *pranayama* (conscious breathing) is a great way of calming the mind, restoring cognitive function, balancing the central nervous system and opening ourselves up to creative problem solving. Chakra Color meditation is a form of Yogic Peace Education that can be done with any age group.

The science of yogic wellness involves an appreciation of the energetic nature of the universe. There are things we cannot see that have enormous impact on the quality of our lives and interactions with one another. If we consider that life is a divine spark (or energy acting on matter), we can easily recognize that there is a force or power potential that contributes to the vital potency that animates us. *Prana* (as indicated in Chapter Three) is life force—the lightest manifestation of matter or the heaviest expression of the spirit—and the accumulation of prana increases our wellness. Yogic Peace Education involves recognizing, generating, conserving and securing prana. If we think of prana as a kind of peace we can readily see that more is good!

Chakras are energy vortices that line the central energetic channel of the human body (the *sushumna*). Especially useful for the introvert in all of us (introverts greatly deplete their stores of prana through speaking and interaction with others) is the benefit of focusing our attention on an activity that restores and replenishes our pranic tanks (if you like) such as coloring. Meditation and Art Therapy are both methods that help us to reduce stress and increase personal wellbeing. The mind can release itself from harmful imaginings through the simple act of coloring because the brain is occupied with equal parts logic and creativity When we use our hands (knitting, cooking, playing music, coloring) we reduce activity in the amygdala—a part of the brain that controls our emotions and the combination of handwork and breath work can assist us to access higher levels of consciousness (Barron and Barron 2013).

Chakra Yoga therapy involves becoming aware of overactive, underactive or blocked chakras. By choosing (either consciously or unconsciously) an image from the following section, learners/facilitators can both appreciate different segments of the energetic body and actively contribute to mental, physical and spiritual wellness. Chakra color meditation involves choosing an image and coloring.

Begin by choosing a surface to color on. Select your medium of color (pens, markers, pencils, crayons) and choose an image to color (the images can be photocopied to any size of paper).

Before the first stroke hits the page simply look at your image and breathe. Take several mindful, deep breaths and permit your conscious and unconscious mind to absorb the graphic image in front of you. Keep breathing. Now you are ready to begin. This is the easy part—without judgment color away.

Use breathing cues—many people hold their breath when they are concentrating on something. Have your participants remain mindful of their breathing during this exercise and encourage them to breath.

It may be useful to ask your "drawers" to consider their own disposition prior to choosing a color page. The following chakra self-assessment exercise may be helpful (but is by no means necessary).

Chakra Self-Assessment

Listen to each question and write down what your thoughts and feeling are after letting the question resonate briefly. You may find your answers take several days to arrive but begin by writing what is here now. Close eyes at the beginning of each question and shift your attention to the location of each chakra.

1st Chakra (Muladhara)

Recently in your life how has your diet been nutritious, satisfying and balanced or poor quality and nutrient poor? Have you had enough warmth and comfort in your life? Do you feel safe?

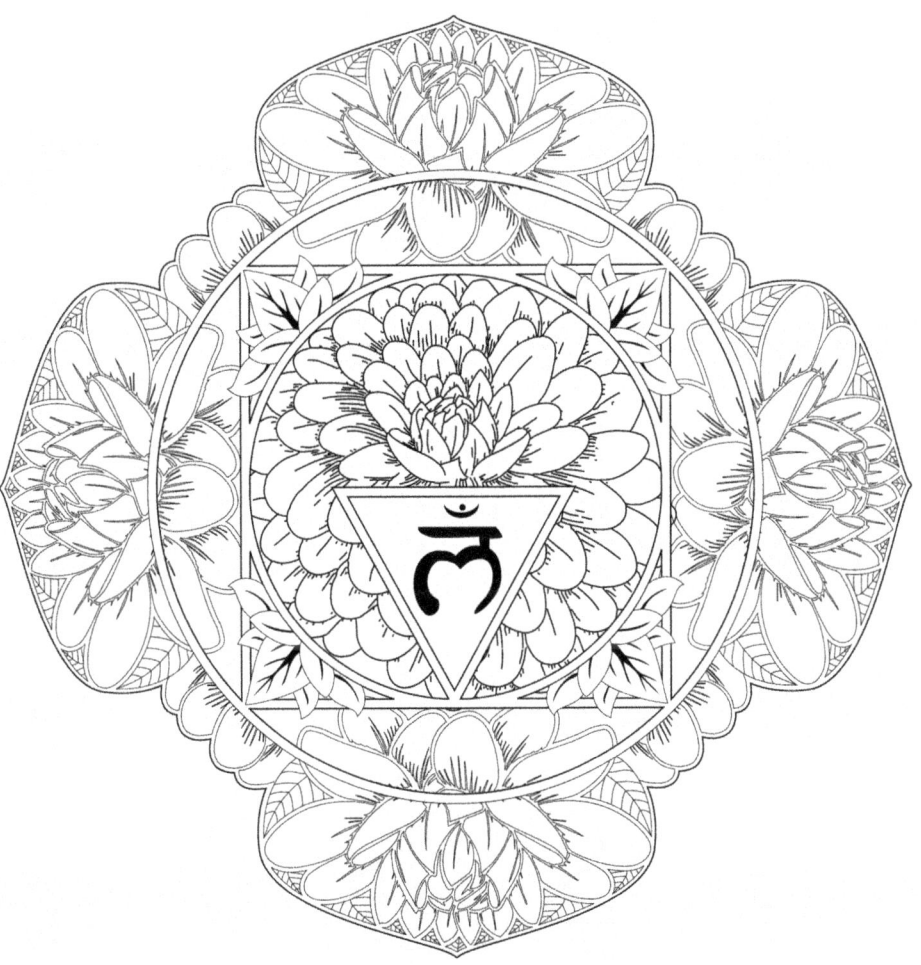

2nd Chakra (*Svadisthana*)

In the last month what have you felt passionate about? Where have you directed your passions? Have you felt true passion? How does creativity manifest in your life?

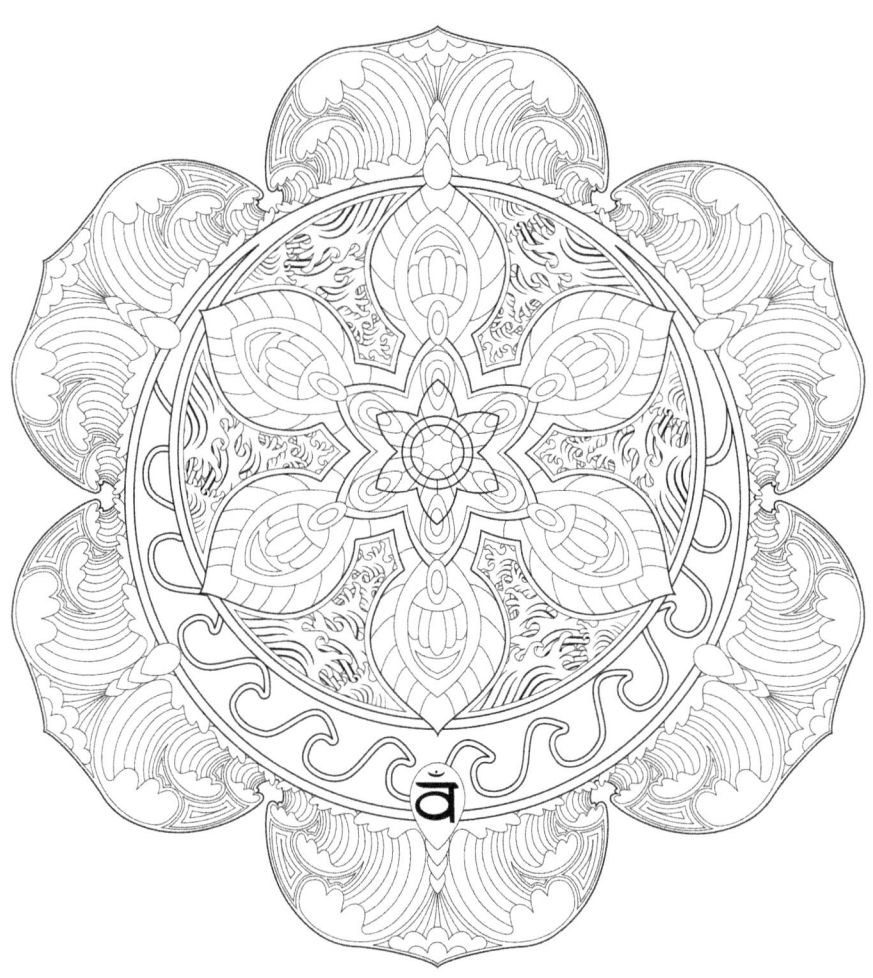

3rd Chakra (*Manipura*)

Does your work in the world (outside of your family) feel satisfying and important to you? Does your work reflect what you value?

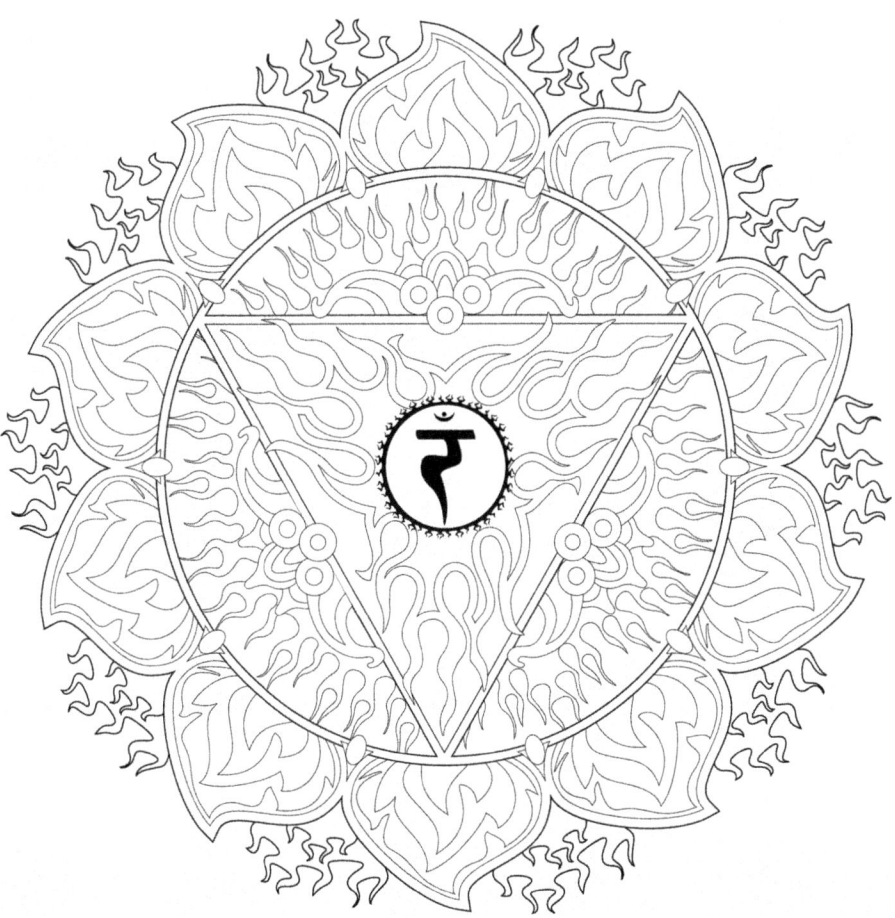

4th Chakra (*Anahata*)

How have you brought compassion into your life recently with family, friends, colleagues and whatever you "touch" with your hands in your life? Do you feel love, feel loving?

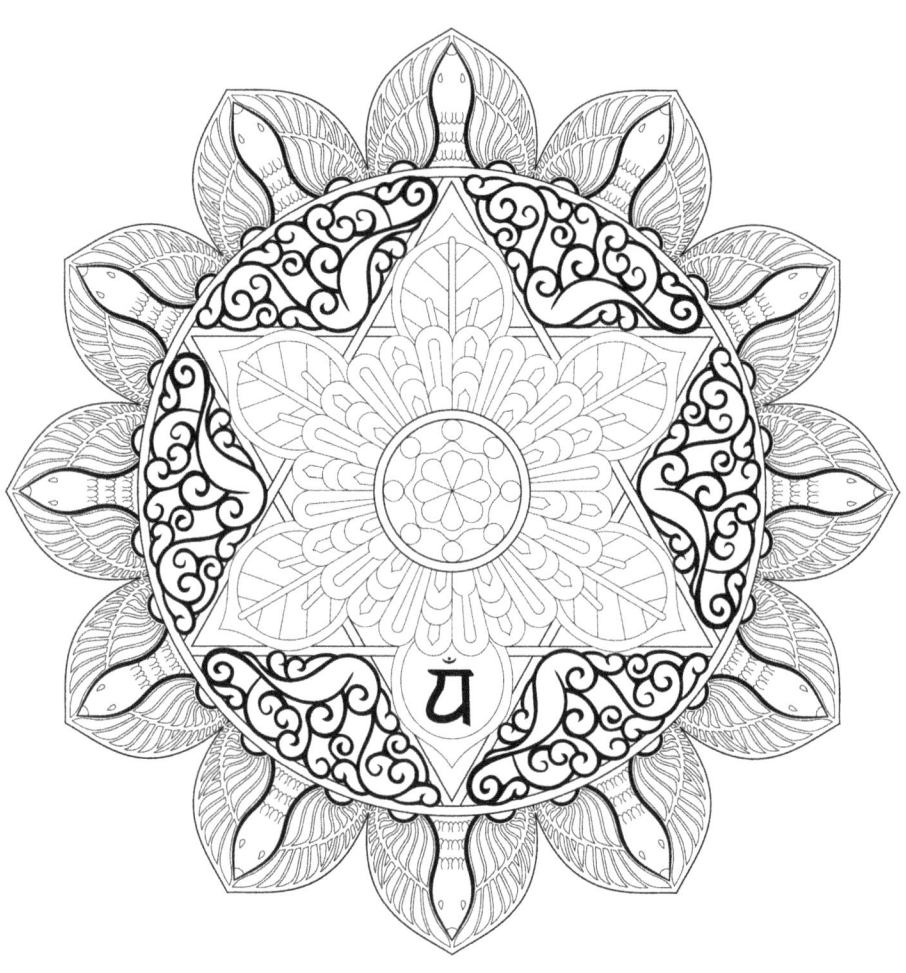

5th Chakra (*Vishuddi*)

In the last few weeks what kind of creative endeavors have you been involved with? Have you expressed your creativity through your voice or through any other modalities? Are you feeling misunderstood?

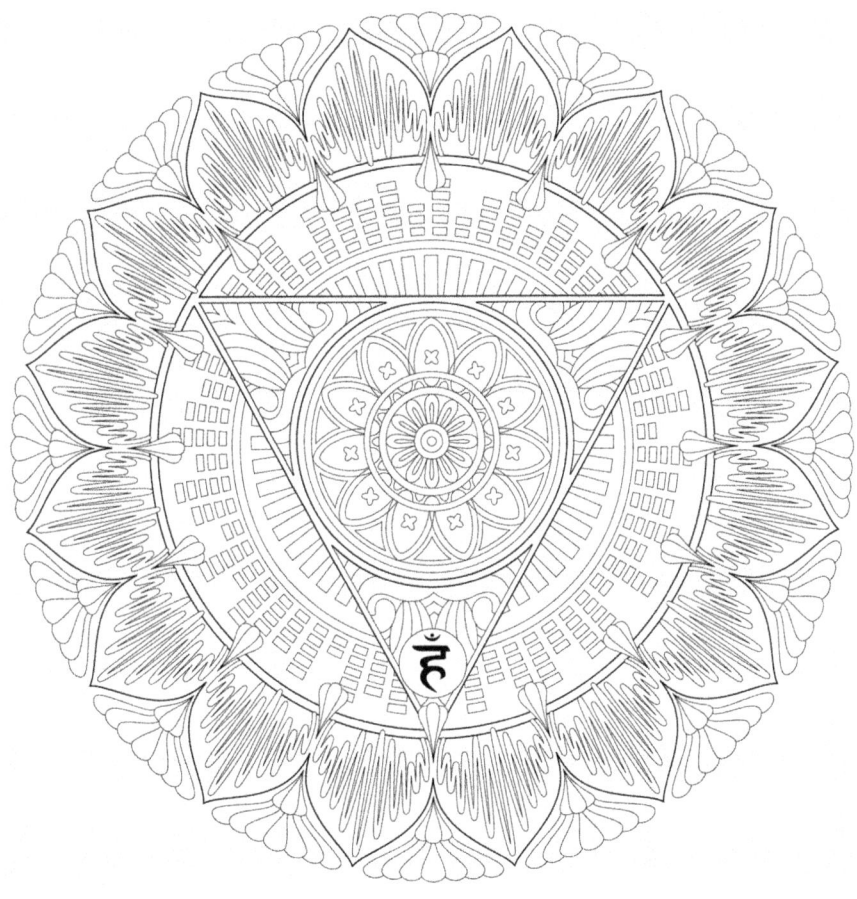

6th Chakra (Ajna)

Recently what have you learned or been studying something new? Do you value knowledge? How has your intuition come into your life?

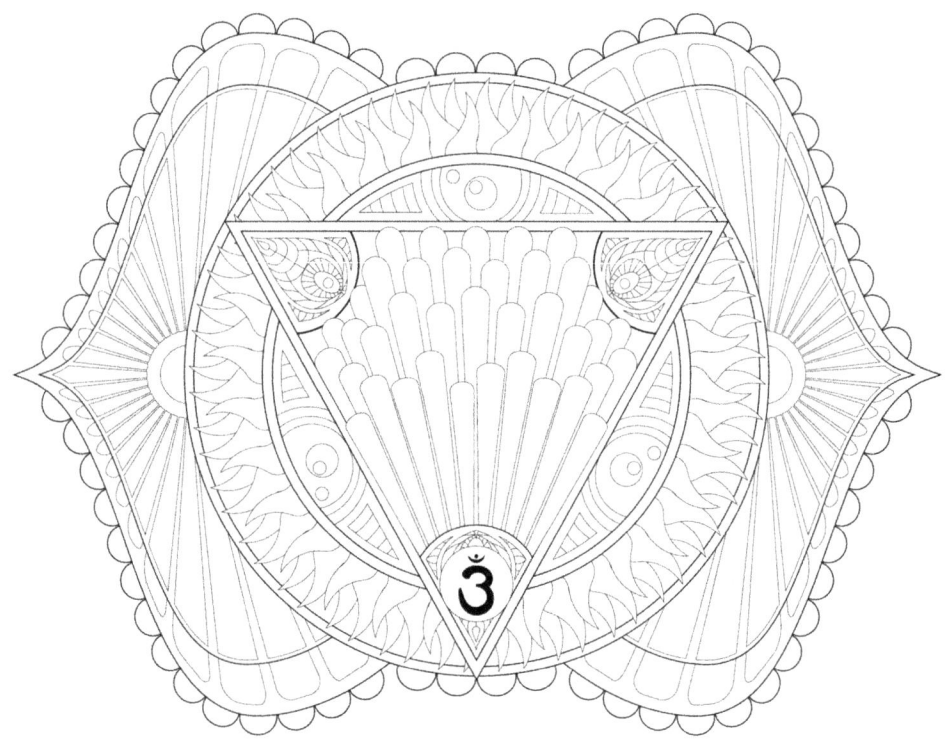

7th Chakra (*Sahasra*)

In the last week or two what have you done spiritually? How have you nourished your spirit? Do you feel connected?

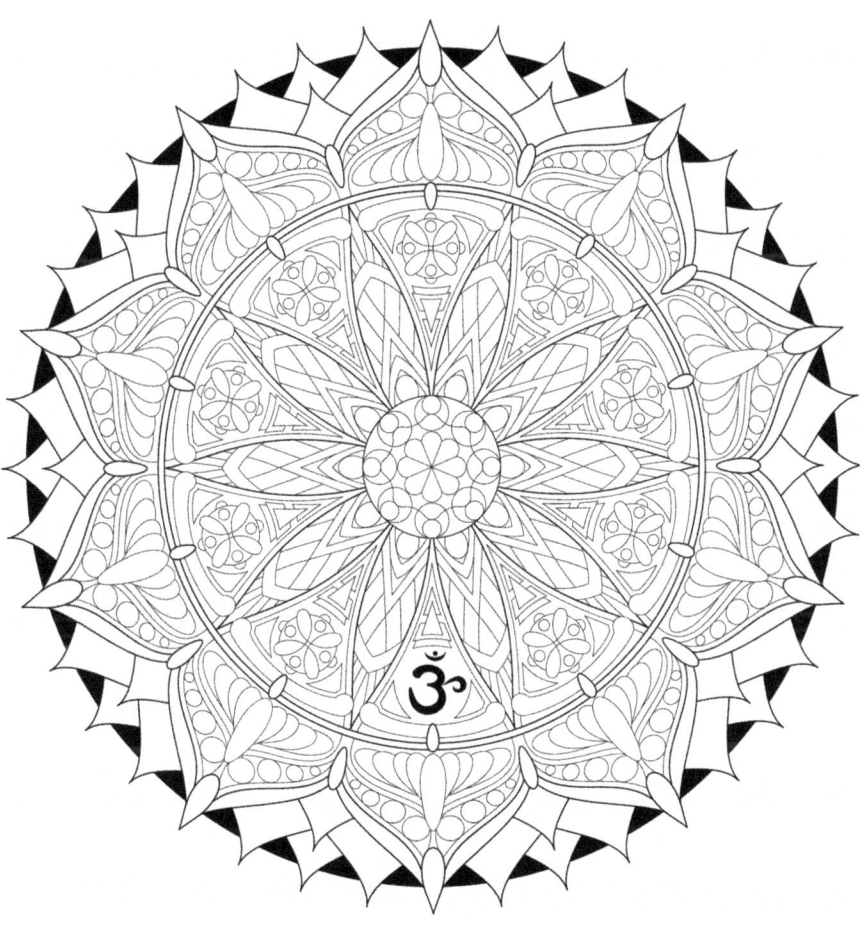

Chapter Notes

Chapter Two

1. Parts of this chapter were previously published in the *Global Journal for Peace Research and Praxis* (Vol. 1[1]) under the title "Cultural Nonviolence: The Other Side of Galtung."

Chapter Three

1. There are several Patanjalis of repute in the ancient manuscripts with some debate as to whether this represents one person or many. It is possible that Patanjali was also a grammarian and mathematician. His work is dated 200 BCE but the practice of Yoga is more ancient, as already discussed. Patanjali's *Yoga Sutras* consists of four chapters: Yoga and its aims, Yoga and its practice, powers, and liberation (*samadhi*) (Prabhavananda 2012, 1). Yoga is codified into eight (*ash*) integrated practices (*tanga*) or limbs.

Chapter Four

1. Energetic does not refer here to energy or effects upon energy levels in the body, but instead to a particular level of existence referred to in Yogic Science as the subtle body (causal body, astral body or, in Kundalini Yoga, the Pranic body), a plane or sphere of existence that is connected to the physical body but extends outward, invisibly to most, to occupy a space that contains pranic (life force) energy and includes energetic organs and pathways called *chakras* and *nadis*.
2. Ontological understandings about the nature of the universe are sometimes very culturally bound. This volume speaks of many alternative conceptualizations and from Yoga a further demarcation exists to further muddy the waters of perception: Kundalini Yoga expands the metaphysical landscape further and utilizes ten bodies (not just three).

Chapter Five

1. *Appropriate* refers to a range of yogic practices—not all of which will be suitable for all practitioners and not all of which will fit into personal lifestyles.

2. *Mantra* refers to the syllable, whereas the action of vocalizing a mantra repeatedly is referred to as chanting.

Chapter Six

1. Spirit in this usage indicates the essential (and invisible) nature of our being and should not be confused with other English-language understandings of spirit that commonly include concepts such as ghosts and souls.
2. Writing about your *worst* trauma can trigger fresh suffering.
3. Writing about the *worst* trauma can trigger fresh suffering.

Bibliography

Abhedananda, Swami. 1967. *Complete works of Swami Abhedananda, vol. 3.* Centenary Publication 1966–1967, Calcutta: Ramakrishna Vedanta Math.
Abhyankar, Ravi. 2015. "Psychiatric thoughts in ancient India." *Mens Sana Monographs*, 13 (1): 59–69.
Adhia, Hasmukh, Nagendra, H. R., Mahadevan, B. 2010. "Impact of Yoga way of life on organizational performance." *International Journal of Yoga*, 3 (2): 55–66.
Allen, Douglas. 2007. "Mahatma Gandhi on Violence and Peace Education." *Philosophy East and West*, 57 (3): 290–310.
Allport, Gordon. W. 1954. *The Nature of Prejudice.* Reading, PA: Addison-Wesley.
Ananthuraman, T.R. 1996. *Ancient Yoga and modern science.* New Delhi: Munishiram Manoharlal Publishing.
Annan, Kofi A. 2005. *In Larger Freedom: Towards development, security and human rights for all: report of the Secretary-General, 2005.* New York: United Nations.
Armstrong, Karen. 2005. *Jerusalem: One city, Three Faiths.* New York: Ballantine Books.
Back, Anthony L., Bauer-Wu, Susan M., Rushton, Cynda H., and Halifax, Joan. 2009. "Compassionate Silence in the Patient-Clinician Encounter: A Contemplative Approach." *Journal of Palliative Medicine*, 12 (12): 1113–1117.
Bajaj, Monisha. 2008. "Critical Peace Education." In *Encyclopedia of Peace Education*, edited by Monisha Bajaj, 127–134. Charlotte, NC: Information Age.
Barnes, Patricia, M., Bloom, Barbara, and Nahin, Richard L. 2009. *Complementary and alternative medicine use among adults and children: United States, 2007.* Hyattsville, MD: U.S. Department of Health and Human Services, Centers for Disease Control and Prevention, National Center for Health Statistics.
Barron, Carrie, and Barron, Alton. 2013. *The Creativity Cure: How to Build Happiness with Your Own Two Hands.* New York: Scribner.
Bar-Tal, Daniel. 2002. "The elusive nature of peace education." In *Peace Education: The Concept, Principles and Practices in the World*, edited by Gavriel Salomon and Baruch Nevo, 27–36. Mahwah, NJ: Lawrence Erlbaum.
Becker, Ina. 2000. "Uses of yoga in psychiatry and medicine." In *Complementary and Alternative Medicine*, edited by Philip R. Muskin, 107–145. Washington, D.C.: American Psychiatric Press.
Benson, Herbert. 1996. *Timeless Healing: The Power and Biology of Belief.* New York: Scribner.
Bharadwaj, Lakshmi K. 1998. "Principled versus Pragmatic nonviolence." *Peace Review*, 10 (1): 79–81.

Bibliography

Bilderbeck, Amy C., Farias, Miguel, Brazil, Inti A., Jakobowitz, Sharon, and Wikholm, Catherine. 2013. "Participation in a 10-week course of yoga improves behavioral control and decreases psychological distress in a prison population." *Journal of Psychiatric Research*, 47 (10): 1438–1445.

Birdee, Gurjeet, Legedza, Anna, Saper, Robert, Bertisch, Suzanne, Eisenberg, David, and Phillips, Russell. 2008. "Characteristics of Yoga Users: Results of a National Survey." *Journal of General Internal Medicine*, 23 (10): 1653–8.

Boal, Augusto. 2000. *Theatre of the Oppressed*. London: Pluto Press.

Boccio, Maddalena, Piccardi, Laura, and Guariglia, Paola. 2015. "The meditative mind: A comprehensive meta-analysis of MRI studies." *BioMed Research International*, 2015: 199–212.

Bolliger, Lindsay, and Want, Hongyu. 2013. "Pedagogy of Nonviolence." *Journal of Curriculum and Pedagogy*, 10 (2): 112–114.

Boulding, Elise. 2000. *Cultures of Peace: The Hidden Side of History*. Syracuse, NY: Syracuse University Press.

Boulding, Kenneth, E. 1978. *Stable Peace*. Austin: University of Texas Press.

Brantmeier, Edward J., and Lin, Jing. 2008. "Toward forging a positive, transformative paradigm for peace education." *Educators as Peacemakers: Transforming education for global peace*, edited by Jing Lin, Edward J. Brantmeier, and Christa Bruhn, xi–2. Charlotte: NC: Information Age Press.

Brantmeier, Edward J. 2007. "Connecting inner and outer peace: Buddhist meditation integrated with peace education." *Journal of Peace Education and Social Justice*, 1 (2): 120–157.

Brefczynski, L. Julie, Lutz, Antoine, Schaefer, Hillary S., Levinson, Daniel B., and Davidson, Richard J. 2007. "Neural correlates of attentional expertise in long-term meditation practitioners." *Proceedings of the National Academy of Science*, 104: 11483–11488.

Brock, Peter. 1999. *Varieties of Pacifism: A Survey from Antiquity to the Outset of the Twentieth Century*. Syracuse, NY: Syracuse University Press.

Brodbeck, S. Pearse. 2007. "Cricket and the Karma Yoga: A comparative study of peak performance." *Sport in Society*, 10 (5): 787–801.

Burley, Mikel. 2014. "A petrification of one's own humanity? Nonattachment and ethics in Yoga traditions." *The Journal of Religion*, 94 (2): 204–228.

Burton, John. 1990. *Conflict: Human Needs Theory*. New York: St. Martin's Press.

Chandrasekaran, Natarajan. 2012. *Principles and practice of Yoga Therapy: A complete guide for learning and practicing Yoga Therapy*, book 1. VHF Publications: Chennai, India.

Clements, Kevin. 2008. "Terrorism: Violent and Non-violent Responses." In *Nonviolence: An Alternative for Defeating Global Terror(ism)*, edited by Senthil Ram and Ralph Summy, 235–256. New York: Nova Science Publishers Inc.

Coates, B.E. 2008. "Modern India's Strategic Advantage to the United States: Her Twin Strengths in Himsa and Ahimsa." *Comparative Strategy*, 27 (2): 33–147. DOI: 10.1080/01495930801944669.

Colcombe, Stanley, and Kramer, Arthur F. 2003. "Fitness effects on the cognitive function of older adults: A meta-analytic study." *Psychological Science*, 14, 125–130.

Collard, Patrizia. 2014. *The Little Book of Mindfulness*. London: Gaia Books.

Condon, Paul, Desbordes, Gaëlle, Miller, Willa B., and Deston, David. 2013. "Meditation increases compassionate responses to suffering." *Psychological Science*, 24 (10): 2125–2127.

Corner, Patricia D. 2009. "Workplace spirituality and business ethics: Insights from an Eastern spiritual tradition." *Journal of Business Ethics*, 85 (3): 377–389.

Bibliography

Côté, Stéphane, DeCelles, Katherine, McCarthy, Julie, Van Kleef, Gerben, and Hideg, Ivona. 2015. "The Jekyll and Hyde of Emotional Intelligence: Emotion-regulation Knowledge facilitates both prosocial and interpersonally deviant behavior." *Psychological Science*, 22 (8): 1073–1080.

Cramer, Holger, Ward, Lesley, Saper, Robert, Fishbein, Daniel, Dobos, Gustav, and Lauche, Romy. 2015. "The Safety of Yoga: A Systematic Review and Meta-Analysis of Randomized Controlled Trials." *American Journal of Epidemiology*, 182 (4): 281–293.

Cramer, Holger, Ward, Lesley, Steel, Amie, Lauche, Romy, Dobos, Gustav and Zhang, Yan. 2016. "Prevalence, Patterns, and Predictors of Yoga Use: Results of a U.S. Nationally Representative Survey: Results of a U.S. Nationally Representative Survey." *American Journal of Preventive Medicine*, 50 (2): 230–235.

Crocker, Jennifer, and Canevello, Amy. 2008. "Creating and undermining social support in communal relationships: the role of compassionate and self-image goals." *Journal of Personality and Social Psychology*, 95 (3): 555–575.

Dasgupta, Surendranath. 1989. *A study of Patanjali*. New Delhi: Motilal Banarsidass Pub., India Council for Philosophical Research.

Dillbeck, Michael C., Cavanaugh, Kenneth L., Glenn, Thomas, and Orme-Johnson, David. 1987. "Consciousness as a field: the Transcendental meditation and TM-Sidhi program and changes in social indicators." *The Journal of Mind and Behaviour*, 8: 67–104.

Ding, Ding, and Stamatakis, Emmanuel. 2014." Yoga practice in England 1997–2008: prevalence, temporal trends, and correlates of participation." *BMC Research Notes*, 7: 172.

Donnelly, Jack. 2003. *Universal Human Rights: In Theory and Practice*, 2nd ed. London: Cornell University Press.

Eifert, George H., and Forsyth, John P. 2008. *The Mindfulness and Acceptance Workbook for Anxiety*. Oakland, CA: New Harbinger Publishers.

Ekman, Paul, Davidson, Richard T., and Frissen, Wallace V. 1990. "The duchenne smile: Emotional expression and brain physiology." *Journal of Personality and Social Psychology*, 58: 342–353.

Englander, Elizabeth K. 2007. *Understanding Violence (3rd Edition)*. Mahwah, NJ: Lawrence Erlbaum Associates.

Felson, Richard. 2009. "Is Violence Natural, Unnatural or r=Rationale?" *The British Journal of Sociology*, 60 (3): 577–585.

Feuerstein, Georg. 2001. *The Yoga Tradition: Its History, Literature, Philosophy and Practice*. Prescott, AZ: Hohm Press.

Field, Tiffany. 2011. "Yoga clinical research review." *Complementary Therapies in Clinical Practice*, 17 (1): 1–8.

Fox, Kieran C., Nijeboer, Savannah, Dixon, Matthew L., Floman, James L., Ellamil, Melissa, Rumak, Samuel P., Sedlmeier, Peter, and Christoff, Kalina. 2014. "Is meditation associated with altered brain structure? A systematic review and meta-analysis of morphometric neuroimaging in meditation practitioners." *Neuroscience and Biobehavioral Reviews*, 43: 48–73.

Freire, Paolo. 2003. *Pedagogy of the Oppressed* (30th Anniversary Edition). New York: Continuum.

Fry, Douglas P. 2007. *Beyond War: The Human Potential for Peace*. New York: Oxford University Press.

Galtung, Johan. 1990. "Cultural Violence." *Journal of Peace Research*, 27 (3): 291–305.

_____. 1996. *Peace by Peaceful Means: Peace and Conflict, Development and Civilization*. London: Sage Publications.

_____. 1969. "Violence, Peace, and Peace Research." *Journal of Peace Research*, 6 (3): 167–191.
Gandhi, Mohandas K. 1983. *The Story of My Experiments with Truth*. New York: Dover Publications.
_____. 1924. "Young India. 4 December." *In Collected Works of Mahatma Gandhi*, 29: 390.
Gard, Tim, Noggle, Jessica, Park, Crystal, Vago, David, and Wilson, Angela. 2014. "Potential self-regulatory mechanisms of Yoga for psychological health." *Frontiers in Human Neuroscience*, 8 (770): 1–21.
Gier, Nicholas F. 2004. *The Virtue of Nonviolence: From Gautama to Gandhi*. Albany: State University of New York.
Gier, Nicholas, and Ranganathan, Shyam. 2007. "A response to Shyam Ranganathan's review of the virtue of nonviolence: From Gautama to Gandhi/ reply to Nicholas Gier." *Philosophy East and West*, 57 (4): 561–566.
Gururaja, Derebail, Harano, Kaori, Toyotake, Ikenaga and Kobayashi, Haruo. 2011. "Effect of yoga on mental health: Comparative study between young and senior subjects in Japan." *International Journal of Yoga*, 4 (1): 7–12.
Haavelsrud, Magnus. 1996. *Education in Developments*. Norway: Arena Publishers.
Harris, Ian. 2004. "Peace education theory." *Journal of Peace Education*, 1 (1), 5–20.
_____, and Morrison, Mary Lee. 2013. *Peace Education*. 3d ed. Jefferson, NC: McFarland.
Heaton, Dennis, Schmidt-Wilk, Jane and Travis, Frederick. 2004. "Constructs, methods and measures for researching spirituality in organizations." *Journal of Organizational Change Management*, 17 (1): 62–82.
Heerey, Erin, and Crossley, Helen. 2013. "Predictive and reactive mechanisms in smile reciprocity." *Psychological Science*, 24 (8): 1446–1455.
Hillman, Charles, H., Belopolsky, Artem V., Snook, Erin M., Kramer, Arthur F., and McAuley, Edward. 2004. "Physical Activity and Executive Control: Implications for Increased Cognitive Health during Older Adulthood." *Research Quarterly for Exercise and Sport*, 75 (2): 176–185.
Holcombe, Kate. 2015. "Does ahimsa mean I can't eat meat?" *Yoga Journal*, 273: 30–33.
Hölzel, Britta K., Ott, Ulrich, Hempel, Hannes, Hackl, Aandrea, Wolf, Katharina, Stark, Rudolf, and Vaitl, Dieter. 2007. "Differential engagement of anterior cingulate and adjacent medial frontal cortex in adept meditators and non-meditators." *Neuroscience Letters*, 421 (1): 16–21.
Hölzel, Britta, Carmody, James, Vangel, Mark, Congleton, C., Yerramsetti, Sita, Gard, Tim, and Lazar, Sara. 2011. "Mindfulness practice leads to increases in regional brain gray matter density." *Neuroimaging*, 191 (1): 36–43.
Howes, Dustin E. 2013. "The Failure of Pacifism and the Success of Nonviolence." *American Political Science Association* 11 (2): 427–446.
Huntington, Samuel P. 1996. *The Clash of Civilizations and the Remaking of World Order*. New York: Simon and Shuster.
Ikai, Saeko, Uchida, Hiroyuki, Suzuki, Takefumi, Tsunoda, Kenichi, Mimura, Masaru, and Fujii, Yasuo. 2013. "Effects of yoga therapy on postural stability in patients with schizophrenia-spectrum disorders: A single-blind randomized controlled trial." *Journal of Psychiatric Research*, 47 (11): 1744–51.
Ikai, Saeko, Suzuki, Takefumi, Uchida, Hiroyuki, Saruta, Juri, Tsukinoki, Keiichi, Fujii, Yasuo and Mimura, Masaru. 2014. "Effects of weekly one-hour Hatha yoga on resilience and stress levels in patients with schizophrenia-spectrum disorders: an eight-week randomized controlled trial." *Journal of Alternative and Complementary Medicine*, 20 (11): 823–30.

Ito, M. 2011. "A history of modern postural yoga in relation to contemporary spirituality culture." *Journal of Religious Studies*, 84: 1255–1256 (in Japanese).

de Jager Meezenbroek, Eltica, Garssen, Bert, van den Berg, Machteld, van Dierendonck, Dirk, Visser, Adriann, and Schaufeli, Wilmar. 2012. "Measuring spirituality as a universal human experience: A review of spirituality questionnaires." *Journal of Religion & Health*, 51: 336–354.

Jefferson-Buchanan, Rachel. 2006. "An introduction to research on Yoga education, Physical Education matters." Retrieved from http://www.ryeuk.org/articles.htm#intro

Joyce, Janine. 2015. "Human spirituality and coming together in peace, looking through two lenses. "PhD: http://hdl.handle.net/10523/5992 OUR Archive—https://ourarchive.otago.ac.nz University of Otago Library—http://www.otago.ac.nz/library

Kabat-Zinn, Jon. 2009. *Wherever You Go, There You Are: Mindfulness Meditation in Everyday Life*. New York: Hyperion.

Kahane, David. 2009. "Learning about obligation, compassion and global justice: The place of contemplative pedagogy." *New Directions for Teaching and Learning*, 118: 49–60.

Kant, Immanuel. 1903. *Perpetual Peace; a philosophical essay, 1795*. London: S. Sonnenschein.

Kauts, Amit, and Sharma, Neelam. 2009. "Effect of Yoga performance in relation to stress." *International Journal of Yoga*, 2 (1): 39–43.

Kim, Gwang Suk, Kim, Eun Gyeong, Shin, Ki Young, Choo, Hee Jung, and Kim, Mi Ja. 2015. "Combined pelvic muscle exercise and yoga program for urinary incontinence in middle-aged women." *Journal of Nursing Science*, 12 (4): 330–339.

Kurlansky, Mark. 2006. *Nonviolence: The History of a Dangerous Idea*. New York: Random House.

Jerath, Ravinder, Edry, John W., Barnes, Vernon A., and Jerath, Vandra. 2006. "Physiology of long pranayamic breathing: neural respiratory elements may provide a mechanism that explains how slow deep breathing shifts the autonomic nervous system." *Med Hypotheses* 67: 566–571.

Landau, Pashupati S., and Gross, John B. 2008. "Low reincarceration rate associated with Ananda Marga Yoga and meditation." *International Journal of Yoga Therapy*, 18 (1): 43–48.

Lederach, John Paul. 1995. *Preparing for Peace*. Syracuse, NY: Syracuse University Press.

_____. 2005. *The Moral Imagination: The Art and Soul of Building Peace*. New York: Oxford University Press.

Lehmann, Dietrich, Faber, Pascal, Tei, Shisea, Pascual-Marqui, Roberto, Milz, Patricia, and Kochi, Keiko. 2012. "Reduced functional connectivity between cortical sources in five meditation traditions detected with lagged coherence using EEG tomography." *NeuroImage*, 60 (2): 1574–1586.

Levy, Becca, Pilver, Corey, Chung, Pil, and Slade, Martin. 2014. "Subliminal Strengthening: Improving older individuals' physical function over time with an implicit-age-stereotype intervention." *Psychological Sciences*, 25(12): 2127–2135.

Lin, Jing. 2006. *Love, Peace, and Wisdom in Education: A Vision for the Education in the 21st Century*. Lanham, MD: Rowman & Littlefield.

Luders, Eileen, Phillips, Owen, Clark, Kristi, Kurth, Florian, Toga, Arthur, and Narr, Katherine. 2012. "Bridging the hemispheres in meditation; Thicker callosal regions and enhanced fractional anisotropy (FA) in long-term practitioners." *NeuroImage*, 61 (1): 181–187.

Luders, Eileen, Clarke, Kristi, Narr, Katherine and Toga, Arthur W. 2011. "Enhanced brain connectivity in long-term meditation practitioners." *NeuroImage*, 57(4): 1308–1316.

Luders, Eileen, Toga, Arthur W., Lepore, Natasha and Gaser, Christian. 2009. "The underlying anatomical correlates of long-term meditation: larger hippocampal and frontal volumnes of grey matter." *NeuroImage*, 45 (3): 672–678.

Lutz, Antoine, Greischar, Lawrence L., Perlman, David, and Davidson, Richard J. 2009. "Bold signal in insula is differentially related to cardiac function during compassion meditation in experts versus novices." *NeuroImage*, 47 (3): 1038–1046.

Marchand, William R. 2014. "Neural mechanisms of mindfulness and meditation: Evidence from neuroimaging studies." *World Journal of Radiology*, 6 (7): 471–479.

Matsushita, Tomoko, and Oka, Takakazu. 2015. "A large-scale survey of adverse events experienced in yoga classes." *BioPsychoSocial Medicine*, 9: 9–14.

McCarthy, Colman. 2002. *I'd Rather Teach Peace*. New York: Orbis Books.

McCraty, Rollin, Barrios-Choplin, Bobo, Rozman, Deborah, Atkinson, Mike, and Watkins, Allen D. 1998. "The impact of a new emotional self-management program on stress, emotions, heart rate variability, DHEA and cortisol." *Integrative Physiological and Behavioural Science*. 33: 151–170.

Merton, Thomas. 1980. *The Nonviolent Alternative: Revised Edition of Thomas Merton on Peace*. Toronto: McGraw-Hill.

Miyata, Hiromitsu, Okanoya, Kazuo, and Kawai, Nobuyuki. 2015. "Mindfulness and psychological status of Japanese Yoga practitioners: a cross-sectional study." *Mindfulness*, 6 (3): 560–571.

Mouffe, Chantal. 1995. "Politics, Democratic Action, and Solidarity." *Inquiry* 38 (1/2): 99–108.

Mulla, Zubin R., and Krishnan, Venkat R. 2006. "Karma Yoga: A conceptualization and validation of the Indian philosophy of work." *Journal of Indian Psychology*, 24 (1/2): 26–43.

Nagashima, Y. 2012. "From 'fitness' to 'retreat'—a cultural history of contemporary yoga." Dissertation. Waseda University (in Japanese).

Nagler, Michael. 2004. *The Search for a Nonviolent Future*. Maui, HI: Inner Ocean.

Nayak, Himanshu, Batra, Sonia, Rachna, Kapoor, Rajendra, Gadhavi, Anand, Solanki, Vyas, Sheetal, and Tiwari, Hemant. 2011. "Prevalence and pattern of stress relaxation practices in Ahmedabad city: A cross-sectional study." *International Journal of Yoga*, 4 (2): 87–92.

Noddings, Nel. 2012. *Peace Education: How We Come to Love and Hate War*. New York: Cambridge University Press.

Orme-Johnson, David W., Alexander, Charles N., Davies, John L., Chandler, Howard M., and Larimore, Wallace E. 1988. "International peace project in the Middle East: The effects of the Maharishi Technology of the unified field." *Journal of Conflict Resolution*, 32: 776–812.

Panduranga, Bhatta C. 2009. "Environment friendly lifestyles: A dialogue with Ancient India." *Decisions*, 36 (3): 103–120.

Paolini, Stefania, Harwood, Jake, and Rubin, Mark. 2010. "Negative intergroup contact makes group memberships salient: Explaining why intergroup conflict endures." *Personality and Social Psychology Bulletin*, 36: 1723–1738.

Parekh, Bhikhu. 1988. "Gandhi's Concept of Ahimsa." *Alternatives: Global, Local, Political*, 13: 195–217.

Penman, Stephen, Cohen, Marc, Stevens, Philip, and Jackson, Sue. 2012. "Yoga in Australia: Results of a national survey." *International Journal of Yoga*, 5 (2): 92–101.

Pennebaker, James W., and Beall, Sandra. 1986. "Confronting a traumatic event:

Toward an understanding of inhibition and disease." *Journal of Abnormal Psychology*, 95 (3): 274–281.
Pettigrew, Ted F. 1998. "Intergroup Contact Theory." *Annual Review of Psychology*, 49: 65–85.
Prabhavananda, Swami. 2012. *Patanjali Yoga sutras*. N.p.: Adhyakrishna Sri Ramakrishna Math.
Prasada, Rama (Trans). 1912. *Patanjalis Yoga sutras with the commentary of Vyasa and the gloss of Vachespati*. New Delhi: Munshiram Mancharlal Publishers.
Radhakrishnan, Sarvepalli. 1974. *Bhagavadgita*. Bombay: Blackie & Son.
Rajagopalachari, Parthsarathi. 2013. *Sahaj Marg Meanderings*. Kolkata, India: Spirituality Hierarchy Publication Trust.
Rajneesh, Osho. 1988. *Turning In*. Berlin: The Rebel Publishing House.
Ram Chandra. 1991. *The Complete Works of Ram Chandra Volume 1*. Kolkata, India: Spiritual Hierarchy Publication Trust.
Rastogi, Ashish, and Pati, Surya P. 2015. "Towards a conceptualization of Karma Yoga." *Journal of Human Values*, 21 (1): 51–63.
Ross, Marc H. 2007. *Cultural Contestation in Ethnic Conflict*. Cambridge: Cambridge University Press.
Roth, John. 2002. *Choosing Against War: A Christian View*. Intercourse, PA: Good Books.
Salomon, Gavriel, and Nevo, Baruch. 1999. "Peace Education: An Active Field in Need for Research," paper presented at a Peace Education Conference, University of Haifa, 7–8 November.
Salzberg, Sharon. 1995. *Loving-kindness: The revolutionary art of happiness*. Boston: Shamballa.
Satyananda, Saraswati. 1966. *Asana Pranayama Mudra Bandha*. Bihar, India: Bihar School of Yoga.
Satyananda, Swami. 1976. *Four chapters on freedom: Commentary on the Yoga sutras of Patanjali*. Munger, India: Yoga Publications Trust.
Sharp, Gene. 1973. *The Politics of Non-violent Action*. Boston: P. Sargent.
_____. 2005. *Waging Non-violent Struggle*. Boston: Hardy Merriman.
Shaw, Malcolm N. 2003. *International Law: Fifth Edition*. Cambridge: Cambridge University Press.
Singh, Kanwaljeet, Bal, Baljinder and Vaz, Wilfred. 2010. "The effect of Suryananaskar yogasana on muscular endurance and flexibility among intercollege yoginis." *Citius Altius Fortius*, 27 (2): 61–67.
Singh, Ramendra, and Singh, Rakesh. 2012. "Karma orientation in boundary spanning sales employees: A conceptual framework and research proposition." *Journal of Indian Business Research*, 4 (3): 140–157.
Singleton, Omar, Britta K. Hölzel, Mark Vangel, Narayan Brach, James Carmody, and Sara W. Lazar. 2014. "Change in Brainstem Gray Matter Concentration Following a Mindfulness-Based Intervention is Correlated with Improvement in Psychological Well-Being." *Frontiers in Human Neuroscience*, 8 (1): 33.
Snauwaert, Dale. 2011. "Social Justice and the philosophical foundations of critical peace education: Exploring Nussbaum, Sen and Freire." *Journal of Peace Education*, 8 (3): 315–331.
Sprecher, Susan, and Fehr, Beverley. 2005. "Compassionate love for close others and humanity." *Journal of Social and Personal Relationships*, 22 (5): 153–158.
Srivastava, Kalpana. 2010. "Human nature: Indian perspective revisited." *Industrial Psychiatry Journal*, 19 (2): 77–81.
Standish, Katerina. 2015. "The Critical Difference of Peace Education." *In Factis Pax: Journal of Peace Education and Social Justice* 9 (1): 27–37.

Bibliography

———. 2014. "Cultural Nonviolence: The other side of Galtung." *Global Journal of Peace Research and Praxis*, 1 (1): 46–54.
Stephan, Maria J., and Chenoweth, Erica. 2008. "Why Civil Resistance Works: The Strategic Logic of Non-violent Conflict." *International Security*, 33 (1): 7–44.
Stephenson, Carolyn M. 2012. "Elise Boulding and peace education: theory, practice, and Quaker faith." *Journal of Peace Education*, 9 (2): 115–126.
Suksohale, Neelam and Phatak, Mrunal. 2012. "Effect of short-term and long-term Brahmakumaris Raja Yoga meditation on physiological variables." *Indian Journal of Physiology Pharmacology*, 56 (4): 388–392.
Suneetha, K. 2013. "Implementing positive values in organisations and education for better living." *Indian Journal of Positive Psychology*, 4 (1): 140–143.
Synott, John. 2005. "Peace education as an educational paradigm: review of a changing field using an old measure." *Journal of Peace Education*, 2 (1): 3–16.
Targ, Russell, and Putchoff, Harold E. 2005. *Mind-Reach: Scientists Look at Psychic Abilities*. Charlottesville, VA: Hampton Roads Publishing.
Terchek, Ronald J. 2001. "Gandhi: Nonviolence and Violence." *Journal of Power and Ethics: An Interdisciplinary Review*, 2 (3): 213–242.
Thomas, John, Jamieson, Graham, and Cohen, Marc. 2014. "Low and then high frequency oscillations of distinct right cortical networks are progressively enhanced by meditation and long term Satyananda Yoga meditation practice." *Frontiers of Human Neuroscience*, 8, 197.
Travis, Fred, and Pearson, Craig. 2000. "Pure consciousness: Distinct phenomenological and physiological correlates of 'consciousness itself.'" *International Journal of Neuroscience*, 100: 1–4.
Trocmé, André. 1961. *Jesus and the Nonviolent Revolution*. Maryknoll, NY: Orbis Books [2003].
UNESCO. 2013. *Culture of Peace and Nonviolence*. Retrieved from: http://www.unesco.org/new/en/bureau-of-strategic-planning/themes/culture-of-peace-and-nonviolence.
Van der Kolk, Bessel A. 2006. "Clinical implications of neuroscience research in PTSD." *Annals of the New York Academy of Sciences*, 1071: 277–293.
Vivekânanda, Swami. 1899. *Vedânta philosophy: Lectures on Raja Yoga*. New York: The Baker and Taylor Company.
Vivekânanda, Swami. 1923. *Raja Yoga conquering the internal nature*. Kolkata: Advaita Ashrama Publication Department.
Volkan, Vamik. 2006. *Killing in the Name of Identity: A Study of Bloody Conflicts*. Charlottesville, VA: Pitchstone.
2006. "Vulnerable Populations: Who Are They?" *American Journal of Managed Care*, 12 (13): 348–352.
Walker, R.B.J. 1988. *One World, Many Worlds: Struggles for a Just World Peace*. Boulder: Lynne Rienner Publishers.
Weaver, Lindy, and Darragh, Amy. 2015. "Systematic Review of Yoga Interventions for Anxiety Reduction Among Children and Adolescents." *The American Journal of Occupational Therapy*, 69 (6): 1–7A.
Weber, Thomas. 2003. "Nonviolence Is Who? Gene Sharp and Gandhi." *Peace & Change*, 28 (2), 250–270. DOI: 10.1111/1468-0130.00261.
Weiss, D. 2006. "*Ahimsâ*—Nonviolence from a Yoga perspective." *Fellowship*, 72 (1–2): 25.
Whicher, Ian. 1998. "The final stage of purification in classical Yoga." *Asian Philosophy*, 8 (2), 85–102.
Wiggins, Joy. 2011. "The search for balance: Understanding and implementing Yoga,

Peace and Democratic Education." *In Factis Pax: Journal of Peace Education and Social Justice*, 5 (2): 216–234.

Wong, Yuk-Lin. 2013. "Returning to Silence, Connecting to Wholeness: Contemplative Pedagogy for Critical Social Work Education." *Journal of Religion and Spirituality in Social Work: Social Thought*, 32:3, 269–285.

Wood, Ernest 1959. *Yoga*. London: Penguin Books.

Index

agápe 18
ahimsa 54, 55, 72, 81
ajna 79
anahata 78
anulom vilom 134
aparigraha 54, 58
asana 45, 53, 61, 84, 131
Ashtanga 32
asteya(m) 54, 57

Bhagavad-gita 46, 52
Bhakti yoga 53, 63
brahmacharya 54, 57
buddhi 46

Chakra coloring meditation 161–69
Chakra yoga 77–79
chakras 76
citta 76
civil disobedience 18
conflict 11–12
conflict resolution education 22
connection 141, 148, 153
consciousness 48, 142, 149, 153
critical consciousness 23
critical peace education 23
cultural nonviolence 31, 35, 39
cultural nonviolence triangle 37
cultural violence 12, 31

development education 22
dharana 53, 84
dhyana 53, 84
direct violence 12
duhkhu 52

education 1
education for sustainability 21

five principles of yogic peace education 116, 136
Freire, Paolo 37
Freireian peace education 26

Galtung, Johan 31
Galtungian peace education 25
Galtung's theory of cultural violence 13
Galtung's violence triangle 38
Gandhi (the Mahatma) Mohandas, K. 16, 18, 32
Gandhian *ahimsa* 32–33, 39
Ghandian peace education 27

Hatha yoga 49, 61, 84
Hatha Yoga Pradipika 62, 134
himsa 39
human rights education 21

ida 77
inner peace 11
integrity 137, 139, 143, 151
international education 21
ishwara pranidhana 61
Islam 17

Jalandhara bandha 63
japa 64
jnana 2, 53
Jnana yoga 53, 65
just peace 11
just war 17

karma 75
Karma yoga 53, 66
King, Martin Luther, Jr. 16
kirtan 93
knowing 82

183

Index

kriya 63, 95

learning 136–7

manas 76
manipura 78
mantra 93
meditation 46, 52
Merton, Thomas 16
metta 132
Montessorian peace education 25
mudra 95
Mula bandha 63
Muladhara 77

nadi shodana 134
nadis 76, 77
nauli 63
negative peace 11
niyama 53, 59, 84
nonviolence 3, 15–19, 139, 144, 151; pragmatic 18; principled 17; *see also ahimsa*; civil disobedience; Gandhian *ahimsa*; nonviolent defense; nonviolent resistance
nonviolent action 35
nonviolent defense 18
nonviolent resistance 18
nonviolent struggle 35

pacifism 11, 15
Parihaka 18
Patanjali 50
peace 7, 10–11
peace education 3, 7
peacebuilding 9, 11
peacekeeping 11
peacemaking 11
perpetual peace 11
pingala 77
positive peace 3, 11
pragmatic nonviolence 34
prana 76, 115
pranayama 53, 61, 84, 127, 134, 161
pranic sheath 76
pratyahara 53
praxis 2, 37

Raja Yoga 53, 54
Reardonian peace education 26

Saint Augustine of Hippo 17
sahasrara 79

samadhi 46, 53
samYoga 52
sankalpa 62
santosha 60, 83
sattvification 73–74
satya(m) 54, 56
satyagraha 18
saucha 59
self-knowledge 2
Sharp, Gene 34
shavasana 62
simplicity 140, 146, 152
social justice 23
stable peace 11
structural violence 12
suicide 3
Surya Namaskar 62, 134
sushumna 77
sustainable peace 11
svadisthana 78
swadhyaya 60
Systems Networks Model 83

tapas 60
Thoreau, Henry 17
The Three Bodies 75
Tolstoy, Leo 16

Uddiyaana bandha 63
Universal Declaration of Human Rights 12

vegetarianism 16, 18
vidya 2
violence 2, 12–15
vishuddhi 79
viYoga 52

world peace 11

yama 32, 53, 55, 84
yantra 93
yoga 3, 45; anatomy 74; and incarcerated populations 109; post-conflict 112; and stress 107; therapy 99, 103
and vulnerable populations 111
Yoga Sutras 32, 53, 62
Yoganidra 62
yogic lifestyle 69
yogic psychology 68
yogic science 2, 48

www.ingramcontent.com/pod-product-compliance
Ingram Content Group UK Ltd.
Pitfield, Milton Keynes, MK11 3LW, UK
UKHW042013140426
5217IPUK00015B/1147